Difficult Airway Management

Edited by

Dr Mansukh Popat

Nuffield Department of Anaesthetics,
John Radcliffe Hospital,
Oxford, UK

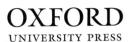

D1492936

OXFORD
UNIVERSITY PRESS

OXFORD
UNIVERSITY PRESS

Great Clarendon Street, Oxford OX2 6DP

Oxford University Press is a department of the University of Oxford.
It furthers the University's objective of excellence in research, scholarship,
and education by publishing worldwide in

Oxford New York

Auckland Cape Town Dar es Salaam Hong Kong Karachi
Kuala Lumpur Madrid Melbourne Mexico City Nairobi
New Delhi Shanghai Taipei Toronto

With offices in

Argentina Austria Brazil Chile Czech Republic France Greece
Guatemala Hungary Italy Japan Poland Portugal Singapore
South Korea Switzerland Thailand Turkey Ukraine Vietnam

Oxford is a registered trade mark of Oxford University Press
in the UK and in certain other countries

Published in the United States
by Oxford University Press Inc., New York

© Oxford University Press, 2009

The moral rights of the author(s) have been asserted
Database right Oxford University Press (maker)

First published 2009

British Library Cataloguing in Publication Data

Data available

Library of Congress Cataloging in Publication Data

Data available

Typeset by Newgen Imaging Systems (P) Ltd., Chennai, India
Printed in Great Britain
on acid-free paper by
Ashford Colour Press Ltd, Gosport, Hampshire

ISBN 978-0-19-955451-5

10 9 8 7 6 5 4 3 2 1

Whilst every effort has been made to ensure that the contents of this book are as complete,
accurate, and-up-to-date as possible at the date of writing. Oxford University Press is not able to give
any guarantee or assurance that such is the case. Readers are urged to take appropriately qualified
medical advice in all cases. The information in this book is intended to be useful to the general
reader, but should not be used as a means of self-diagnosis or for the prescription of medication.

Contents

Preface

The establishment of optimal oxygenation and ventilation of the patient's lungs is a fundamental goal of every anaesthetic and essential to patient safety. Anaesthetists achieve this by a variety of tools and techniques. Whilst this is uneventful in the majority of cases, difficulties do arise. The consequences of failure may be catastrophic to both the patient and the anaesthetist.

Much progress has been made in the understanding of causative factors and management of difficult airway scenarios in the last 15 years. Guidelines from various national societies have played a pivotal role in defining a structured approach for these scenarios and industry has responded by the introduction of new equipment.

It is therefore important for the clinical anaesthetist, faced with airway difficulties on a regular basis, to approach its management in a structured, practical fashion. There are many approaches to difficult airway management. In this book we have used one that is familiar to us and one that we routinely teach. Our approach is based on a scheme based on the 5 'P's – Preoperative assessment, Planning, Procedures, Post procedures and Publicity. The scheme is used to describe management of scenarios – the anticipated (with and without airway obstruction) and unanticipated (can't intubate – can and can't ventilate) difficult airway. Some special situations relating to patient (e.g. paediatrics, obstetrics, obesity) and environmental factors (e.g. emergency room) are covered separately. Separate chapters describing basic anatomical and physiological aspects, as well as the latest equipment and training aspects, ensure that all aspects of the subject are covered.

Each chapter is written in a concise, structured way and includes key points and a further reading list. The emphasis is to describe the approach in a simple, easy to understand and practical way; where appropriate techniques are described in detail. All the authors are members of the Oxford Region Airway Group (ORAG). This group was formally convened in September 2004, to provide a forum for anaesthetists in the Oxford Region to advance airway related training, audit and research.

In a book of this size, it is impossible to include photos of techniques, so vital in disseminating messages about difficult airway management. A unique feature of this book is the inclusion of photos, slides and video clips on the ORAG website – www.orag.co.uk/book. The reader is prompted to refer to the website in the appropriate sections of each chapter. These will be updated in future as techniques evolve.

PREFACE

I am extremely grateful to those colleagues who have contributed to our clinical experience in dealing with 'difficult airway' patients and in helping us set up our training programme. Many have also made helpful suggestions on the manuscript of this book.

Dr Mansukh Popat
Consultant Anaesthetist,
Nuffield Department of Anaesthetics,
John Radcliffe Hospital,
Oxford

Contributors

Imran Ahmad
Specialist Registrar,
Nuffield Department
of Anaesthetics,
John Radcliffe Hospital,
Oxford, UK

Stuart W. Benham
Consultant Anaesthetist,
Nuffield Department of Anaesthetics,
John Radcliffe Hospital,
Oxford, UK

Imogen Davies
Specialist Registrar,
Nuffield Department of Anaesthetics,
John Radcliffe Hospital,
Oxford, UK

Ravi Dravid
Consultant Anaesthetist,
Kettering General Hospital,
Kettering, UK

Chris Frerk
Consultant Anaesthetist,
Department of Anaesthesia,
Northampton General Hospital,
Northampton, UK

Mike Goodwin
Consultant Anaesthetist,
Department of Anaesthesia,
Northampton General Hospital,
Northampton, UK

Rehana Iqbal
Consultant Anaesthetist,
St George's Hospital,
London, UK

Atul Kapila
Consultant Anaesthetist,
Royal Berkshire Hospital,
Reading, UK

Gene Lee
Specialist Registrar,
Nuffield Department of
Anaesthetics,
John Radcliffe Hospital,
Oxford, UK

Alexander Marfin
Consultant Anaesthetist,
Nuffield Department of
Anaesthetics,
John Radcliffe Hospital,
Oxford, UK

David Mason
Consultant Paediatric Anaesthetist,
Nuffield Department of
Anaesthetics,
John Radcliffe Hospital, Oxford, UK

Hamid Manji
Consultant Anaesthetist,
Milton Keynes General Hospital,
Milton Keynes, UK

Ben Maxwell
Consultant Anaesthetist,
Great Western Hospital,
Swindon, UK

Sara McDouall
Specialist Registrar,
Nuffield Department of
Anaesthetics,
John Radcliffe Hospital, Oxford, UK

CONTRIBUTORS

Kawshala Peiris

Specialist Registrar,
Department of Anaesthesia,
Northampton General Hospital,
Northampton, UK

Jaideep J. Pandit

Consultant Anaesthetist,
Nuffield Department
of Anaesthetics,
John Radcliffe Hospital,
Oxford, UK

Mansukh Popat

Consultant Anaesthetist,
Nuffield Department
of Anaesthetics,
John Radcliffe Hospital,
Oxford, UK

Mridula Rai

Consultant Anaesthetist,
Nuffield Department
of Anaesthetics,
John Radcliffe Hospital,
Oxford, UK

Jairaj Rangasami

Consultant Anaesthetist,
Wexham Park Hospital,
Slough, UK

Shaun Scott

Consultant Anaesthetist,
Nuffield Department
of Anaesthetics,
John Radcliffe Hospital,
Oxford, UK

Jenny Thompson

Consultant Anaesthetist,
Nuffield Department
of Anaesthetics,
John Radcliffe Hospital,
Oxford, UK

Abbreviations

AFI	Awake Fibreoptic Intubation
AIC	Aintree Intubation Catheter
ASA	American Society of Anesthesiologists
ATLS	Advanced Trauma and Life Support
BURP	Backward, upward and rightward pressure
CEMACH	Confidential Enquiry into Maternal and Child Health
CICV	Can't intubate can't ventilate scenario
CP	Cricoid pressure
CPAP	Continuous positive airway pressure
CS	Conscious sedation
CSE	Combined spinal epidural
CT	Computerised tomography
DAS	Difficult Airway Society
DL	Direct laryngoscopes
ECG	Electrocardiogram
ENT	Ear, Nose and Throat
ETVC	Endo-tracheal ventilation catheter
FRC	Functional residual capacity
IL	Indirect laryngoscopes
ILMA	Intubating laryngeal mask airway
LMA	Laryngeal mask airway
MAD	Mucosal Atomizer Device
MRI	Magnetic resonance imaging
NAP 4	4th National Audit Project
NPPO	Negative pressure pulmonary oedema
OELM	Optimal external laryngeal manipulation
OMI	Oxford Medical Illustration
OSA	Obstructive sleep apnoea
PER	Pre-Extubation Review

Chapter 1

Difficult airway: definitions, incidence and consequences

Rehana Iqbal and Atul Kapila

Key points

- Precise definitions of difficult airway scenarios are lacking
- For this reason the exact incidence of difficult airway scenarios is unknown
- The consequences of lack of oxygenation due to difficulty or failure with face mask, supraglottic device, tracheal tube or transtracheal device can be catastrophic
- Human behaviour is an important contributor to airway morbidity.

The prime goal in airway management is to SAFELY provide oxygenation and ventilation. Morbidity and mortality result when oxygenation cannot be provided. This may occur if there is difficulty or failure with face mask, supraglottic device, tracheal tube and transtracheal devices. This is an infrequent occurrence.

This chapter will describe some of the definitions used for difficult airways and how these relate to current clinical practice, the limitations of the data available for determining the incidences of difficulty and the consequences of poor management.

1.1 Definitions

Upper airway patency is usually maintained in three ways by anaesthetists. The first is via a natural airway using a face mask with anatomical opening manoeuvres. The second is via a supraglottic device and the third is via a tracheal tube. Problems may occur with one or more of these techniques.

The dictionary defines difficult as that which requires 'effort or skill to do'. In the context of the 'difficult' airway within anaesthesia this meaning is not very useful as management of any normal airway also requires specific skills. The question is at what point should difficulty be defined?

1.1.1 **Difficult airway**

There are several definitions for the difficult airway and no consensus in the literature. The most commonly used definition is that described by the American Society of Anesthesiologists Task Force on management of the difficult airway:

> *A difficult airway is defined as the clinical situation in which a conventionally trained anaesthetist experiences difficulty with mask ventilation, difficulty with tracheal intubation or both.*

This definition does not take account of the use of supraglottic devices. To reflect current practice one could modify the above definition:

> *A difficult airway is the clinical situation in which a conventionally trained anaesthetist experiences difficulty with face mask ventilation, difficulty with supraglottic device ventilation, difficulty with tracheal intubation or all three.*

The above definitions take into account only the 'technical' aspects of airway management. Safe airway management is an inter play between patient factors, clinical settings and skills, experience and behaviour of the individual anaesthetist. In this context, perhaps an appropriate definition for the 'difficult airway' would be:

> *The clinical scenario when safe oxygenation and ventilation cannot be achieved in the **desired way** with the use of an individual's usual practice.*

There are two possibilities that of 'failure' or 'difficulty'. Failure has a clear endpoint in that the attempt is abandoned and the goal is not achieved. A description of difficulty is vaguer as will be outlined with the definitions below. Failure does not necessarily mean that the patient has come to harm for example a failed intubation managed appropriately with oxygenation and ventilation.

1.1.2 **Intubation**

Difficulty in inserting a tracheal tube into the trachea may occur as a result of a poor laryngoscopic view and/or difficulty in passing the tracheal tube through the glottis.

1.1.2.1 *Failed intubation*

This is the inability to place a tracheal tube in the trachea. The incidence is described as 1:2230 in the general population and 1:750-1:280 in the obstetric population. Although the endpoint is clear there is no universal agreement of how many attempts are allowed before abandoning and labelling an intubation as 'failed'. There is no inclusion also of the techniques attempted for intubation. New devices for facilitating intubation are constantly emerging on the market. Individual anaesthetists will have variable experience and skill with these devices. Those who possess particular skills with video-assisted laryngoscopy or fibreoptic equipment may intubate a patient in whom intubation is not possible with conventional laryngoscopy. Technically a failed intubation has not occurred. Therefore when reporting failed intubation the definition would be more meaningful clinically *if mention is made of the number of attempts made with each device and the intubation technique or device which has resulted in failure was included.*

1.1.2.2 *Difficult intubation*
There is no universally accepted definition. In 1993 the American Society of Anesthesiologists defined this as 'the proper insertion of an endotracheal tube with conventional laryngoscopy that requires more than three attempts and/or more than 10 minutes. This definition had clear shortcomings and has been replaced in 2003 by:

Tracheal intubation requires multiple attempts, in the presence or absence of tracheal pathology.

An alternative definition suggested by the Canadian Task Force is when an experienced laryngoscopist, using direct laryngoscopy:

1. requires more than two attempts with same blade or a change in the blade
2. or requires an adjunct to a direct laryngoscope such as a bougie
3. or uses an alternative device/technique following failed intubation with direct laryngoscopy.

This definition is more appropriate as it reflects events which are likely to occur in clinical practice.

1.1.2.3 *Difficult laryngoscopy*
This is when it is not possible to visualise any portion of the vocal cords after multiple attempts at conventional laryngoscopy.

This would equate to a Cormack and Lehane grade 3 or 4 and is a laryngoscopic view associated with difficulty in intubation. The incidence of a grade 3 Cormack and Lehane view is between 1–2%. Although the experience of the anaesthetist is relevant ANY difficult laryngoscopy should be taken seriously and choosing a previously failed anaesthetic plan for subsequent anaesthetics is a risky strategy.

1.1.2.4 *Optimal/best attempt at laryngoscopy*
There are several limitations of the above definitions for difficult intubation and difficult laryngoscopy.

a) Firstly a definition based on the number of laryngoscopic attempts and time is illogical, as an experienced anaesthetist may identify a difficult intubation at the first attempt and within 30 seconds and decide to intubate using an alternative technique.

b) Current guidelines for the management of a difficult intubation are aimed at avoiding harm to the patient with the focus on oxygenation, ventilation and importantly minimization of intubation attempts to avoid airway trauma. For this reason anaesthetists should achieve their best attempt at laryngoscopy as early as possible and if this fails then an alternative technique should be employed for intubation.

c) Intubation is dependant on laryngoscopic view and ability to pass a tracheal tube through the glottis. If optimal attempt at direct laryngoscopy is undertaken this would reduce, although not exclude, operator variability.

The concept of optimal or best attempt at laryngoscopy was introduced by Benumof to overcome the above limitations and would include:

1. Performance by a reasonably experienced anaesthetist
2. Use of optimal sniffing position
3. Use of optimal external laryngeal manipulation (OELM). This will push the larynx posteriorly and cephalad and can reduce the incidence of a grade 3 laryngoscopic view from 9% to 1.3%.
4. One change in the blade length
5. One change in the type of the blade

Airway morbidity is associated with repeated attempts at airway instrumentation with the same or different device and for this reason optimizing direct laryngoscopy avoids unnecessary intubation attempts.

1.1.3 **Bag mask ventilation**

1.1.3.1 *Difficult face mask ventilation*

The ASA definition in 1993 was:

Difficult bag mask ventilation is the situation when it is not possible for the unassisted anaesthesiologist to maintain an oxygen saturation greater than 90% using 100% inspired oxygen and positive pressure ventilation in a patient with a pre-operative saturation greater than 90% before anaesthetic intervention

Or

It is not possible for the unassisted anaesthesiologist to prevent or reverse signs of inadequate ventilation during positive pressure mask ventilation.

This definition was changed in 2003:

a) It is not possible for the anaesthesiologist to provide adequate face mask ventilation due to one or more of the following:
Inadequate mask seal, excessive gas leak or excessive resistance to ingress or egress of gas.

b) Signs of inadequate face mask ventilation include absent or inadequate chest movement, absent or inadequate breath sounds, cyanosis, gastric air entry or dilatation, decreasing or inadequate oxygen saturation, decreasing or inadequate exhaled carbon dioxide, absent or inadequate spirometric measures of exhaled gas flow and haemodynamic changes associated with hypoxemia or hypercarbia.

The incidence ranges between 0.08%–5%. This variable quoted incidence is due to differences in defining what constitutes 'difficult'.

There are degrees of difficulty (Figure 1) and ultimately failure to bag mask ventilate.

Figure 1.1 Degrees of difficulty in face mask ventilation

(i)	(ii)	(iii)	(iv)

(i) One person bag mask ventilation with chin lift +/- jaw thrust
(ii) Above + oropharyngeal or nasopharyngeal airway or both
(iii) Above + assistant to squeeze bag or assistant to provide jaw thrust/face mask seal whilst primary anaesthetist maintains chin lift/face mask seal and squeezes bag
(iv) Anaesthetist plus two assistants: one to squeeze bag and other to provide jaw thrust/face mask seal.

1.1.3.2 *Failed bag mask ventilation*

This is the failure of optimal/best attempt at bag mask ventilation, i.e. the situation where optimal airway opening manoeuvres, head positioning, the use of oral and/or nasopharyngeal airways and assistance fail.

1.1.4 **Laryngeal mask airway**

The laryngeal mask airway has been recommended as a rescue device for ventilation when face mask ventilation and/or intubation have failed. For this reason it has a very important role in airway management and its use has been included in difficult airway guidelines.

1.1.4.1 *Difficult laryngeal mask airway*

This is when the laryngeal mask airway is unable to provide adequate airway patency, oxygenation and ventilation despite correct selection of the laryngeal mask size and provision of optimal airway opening manoeuvres when inserted.

The signs of inadequate ventilation with laryngeal mask airway are similar to those described for inadequate face mask ventilation.

1.1.4.2 *Failure of the laryngeal mask airway*

This is the inability for the laryngeal mask to maintain airway patency and allow the provision of oxygenation and ventilation. This is an uncommon occurrence and incidences have been reported between 0.19 and 0.4% in the normal population.

Comparison between studies is difficult due to the lack of uniformity amongst definitions with regards to number of attempts before failure concluded. Failure occurs due to failed placement or an inadequate seal. Airway morbidity is associated with repeated attempts and generally no more than three attempts, with changes in insertion technique and/or size of laryngeal mask would be made. Anecdotal data suggest that the incidence of difficulties and/or failure is higher with the single use devices.

1.2 **Incidences**

The exact incidences of difficult airways are unknown. The reasons for this are

    a) Lack of uniformity of definitions. For this reason incidences reported for 'difficulty' tend to have a wider range unlike 'failures' which have a clearer endpoint.

b) Population differences. Most of available data does not distinguish between failures in patients with anatomically 'normal' airways and those with predicted difficulty. For example it would be useful to know the incidence of failed laryngeal mask airway in the scenario where difficulty with alternative airway management techniques has occurred.

c) Numbers are dependant on operator reporting. In the absence of mandatory requirements difficult airways may be encountered and not reported.

d) There are no denominators. For example the American Society of Anaesthetists closed claims database has been the best source for data. Likewise in the UK the triennial maternal reports give numbers of deaths due to failed intubation. In both sources the denominator is unknown and hence the exact incidence is unknown.

Table 1.1 summarizes the incidence of various scenarios of difficult airway in the general population. The data are taken from various sources and are intended to give the reader just an idea of the extent of the problem rather than accurate figures.

1.2.1 **4th National Audit Project**

The 4th National Audit Project (NAP 4) seeks to increase our knowledge of the frequency and nature of major airway complications occurring in UK hospitals. This ambitious project is being conducted jointly by the Royal College of Anaesthetists (RCoA) and the Difficult Airway Society (DAS). Between September 2008 and August 2009 NAP 4 will determine the incidence of major complications of airway management in UK anaesthetic practice. To achieve this objective a snapshot of current airway management techniques in use (providing the denominator) will be undertaken for two weeks, and details of major complications (death, brain damage, emergency surgical airway, unanticipated ICU/HDU admission) will then be prospectively collected over one year (to provide a numerator). Airway problems with these endpoints are likely to be:

• difficult or delayed intubation;
• failed intubation;
• failed mask ventilation (including supraglottic airways);
• CICV – the can't intubate can't ventilate scenario.

Table 1.1 Incidence of difficult airway in the general population	
Difficult laryngoscopy (grades 3–4)	10%
Difficult intubation	1%
Failed intubation	0.05%
Difficult bag mask ventilation	0.08–5%
Failed ventilation	0.01–0.03%
Difficult LMA	4.1%
Failed LMA insertion	0.19–0.4%

1.3 **Consequences**

The management of 'difficult airway' more often results in a safe outcome for the patient even in the most difficult circumstances. Morbidity and even mortality does however occur and has been a cause of concern to anaesthetists for generations. Minor morbidity consists of trauma to structures in and around the mouth and teeth. More serious injuries to pharynx, larynx, trachea and even the oesophagus have been described. The ASA closed claims analysis showed the most frequent sites of injury were the larynx (33%), pharynx (19%), and oesophagus (18%). Complications related to pharyngolaryngeal perforation may present early with emphysema or later with mediastinitis which highlights the importance of monitoring these patients in an appropriate environment with a high index of suspicion for late complications. However it is the consequences of failure to provide oxygenation during difficult airway management that is the real cause of concern. This can lead to brain death and even death of the patient.

Of the 34 % respiratory claims in the ASA closed claims project, around 6% were due to difficulties in intubation. Further analysis showed that difficulty was anticipated in around 48% of these patients. Despite this the airway management strategy included multiple attempts eventually resulting in a can't ventilate scenario in around two thirds of these patients. 'The most common scenario… was the development of progressive difficulty in ventilating via mask between persistent and prolonged failed intubation attempts. It is clear that this scenario could have been avoided in most cases.

The last two reports from the Confidential Enquiry into Maternal and Child Health (CEMACH) have shown an increase in maternal deaths directly attributable to anaesthesia with respiratory events featuring as the major contributor either in the form of oesophageal intubation, hypoventilation or respiratory failure. The definitions of failed and difficult intubation based on number of attempts could lead to harm as it implies that more than three attempts at intubation can and perhaps should be made. It is clear from analysis of claims that the focus should be on provision of oxygenation and ventilation rather than repeated attempts with the original airway management strategy.

So why do anaesthetists choose a high risk airway management strategy? Lack of technical skills especially performing some advanced techniques such as awake intubation is a fundamental problem. The contribution of 'non technical' factors such as human behaviour, lack of documentation/availability of information regarding previous difficulties and the environment in which airway management is undertaken is increasingly recognised. This is where risk can and should be minimised.

Some of the reasons for this risky behaviour and technical failure are summarized below

    a) The first is that anaesthetists have knowledge of the fact that failure to oxygenate a patient is a rare occurrence and that there are no good bedside tests for predicting this (Chapter 4). In the majority of cases where difficulty is anticipated no problems occur leading to reinforcement of a high risk approach.

b) There is currently a variety of airway equipment on the market. This can lead to an inappropriate airway management strategy. The reasons for this may be due to lack of confidence and experience with alternative techniques and equipment or due to lack of understanding of the role of these new devices in individual cases. This is partly due to the lack of studies which evaluate alternative techniques in the anticipated difficult airway.

c) Delayed recognition of severity of difficulty. In most cases where difficulty is encountered commonly used adjuncts are successful and for this reason there may be a misplaced confidence in these with further delay in provision of oxygenation.

d) Denial that failure has occurred. Once failure to oxygenate has occurred behaviour is likely to be reactive. For this reason alternative plans must be decided on prior to initiating the original airway management plan.

e) Communication and documentation. At present anaesthetists are reliant on information from patient, general practitioner or old notes. There is a lack of local or regional databases for patients with difficult airways although these are emerging. The use of medic alert bracelets may be appropriate.

f) Environment. Anaesthesia undertaken in the non elective setting is potentially more risky. This is possibly one of the contributing factors in the greater incidence of failed intubation in the obstetric population. Time pressure in the patient presenting for urgent surgery is likely to result in inadequate planning with a resulting poor airway management strategy.

Problems with airway management can occur at any point from induction to recovery. When difficulty has been encountered the importance of monitoring post event cannot be overemphasized. The introduction of guidelines for management of difficult airways is felt to be contributory to the decrease in number of claims made for brain damage and death in American closed claims analysis. Although problems with airway management intra-operatively and at emergence are less frequent there has been no reduction seen in their contribution to overall airway morbidity. Strategies for extubation following problems at induction are potentially an area which would require further work.

The number of patients presenting with potentially challenging airways is increasing. This is partly due to improvements in treatment of airway and facial pathology with later presentation for unrelated surgery. An increase in airway catastrophes can only be avoided by greater emphasis on education, acquirement of a small number of alternative techniques, better communication/ documentation of problems encountered and further work on planning of the entire perioperative pathway for airway management.

Further Reading

American Society of Anaesthetists Task Force on Management of the Difficult Airway. Practice guidelines for Management of the Difficult Airway. *Anesthesiology* 1993; **78**: 597–602.

American Society of Anaesthetists Task Force on Management of the Difficult Airway. Practice guidelines for Management of the Difficult Airway. An updated report. *Anesthesiology* 2003; **95**: 1269–77.

Benumof JL. Management of the difficult airway: with special emphasis on awake tracheal intubation. *Anesthesiology* 1991; **75**: 1087–110.

Brimacombe J. Analysis of 1500 laryngeal mask uses by one anaesthetist in adults undergoing routine anaesthesia. *Anaesthesia* 1996; **51**: 76–80.

Cheney FW, Posner KL, Caplan RA. Adverse respiratory events infrequently leading to malpractice suits. A closed claims analysis. *Anesthesiology* 1991 **75**: 932–9.

Cheney FW, Posner KL, Lee LA, Caplan RA, Domino KB. Trends in anesthesia-related death and brain damage: A closed claims analysis. *Anesthesiology*. 2006; **105**: 1081–6.

Crosby ET, Cooper RM, Diyghlas MJ et al. The unanticipated difficult airway with recommendations for management. *Can J Anaesth* 1998; **45**: 757–76.

Domino KB, Posner KL, Caplan RA, Cheney FW. Airway Injury during Anaesthesia, *Anesthesiology* 1999; **91**: 1703–11.

Henderson JJ, Popat MT, Latto IP, Pearce AC. Difficult Airway Society guidelines for management of the unanticipated difficult intubation. *Anaesthesia* 2004; **59**: 675–94.

Saving mother's lives: confidential enquiry into maternal and child health 2003–2005. http://www.cemach.org.uk/Publications/CEMACH-Publications/Maternal-and-Perinatal-Health.aspx

Vergehese C, Brimacombe JR. Survey of laryngeal mask airway usage in 11,910 patients: safety and efficacy for conventional and non conventional usage. *Anesthesia and Analgesia* **82**: 129–33.

Chapter 2

Difficult airway management: general principles

Mansukh Popat

Key points

- Difficult airway algorithms are not intended to be used as wall charts that could be accessed when problems occur but are designed as a tool to aid the anaesthetists' decision-making skills
- The guidelines form the basis of structured training in difficult airway management
- The management of difficult airway is best understood by and discussed as a 'scenario' based scheme
- Managing each scenario clinically is best achieved by the 5 'P's approach

The 5 'P' are: **P**reoperative airway assessment, **P**lanning, **P**rocedures (techniques used to execute the plan), **P**ost procedure (extubation and follow up) and **P**ublicity (telling others).

2.1 Introduction

In the 1990s, analysis of closed claims data in the US revealed that airway related mishaps were a significant source of anaesthetic malpractice claims; most of these events were preventable and improved strategies for management of difficult airway were urgently required. In response, the American Society of Anesthesiologists (ASA) produced the document 'Practice guidelines for management of the difficult airway', first published in 1993 (revised in 2003). This landmark document was the first time that a national recommendation based on current evidence and consensus opinion was made which allowed for management of the difficult airway in a structured way. Although these recommendations are not a 'standard of care' in the true sense, they were the first step in revolutionizing the management and training of difficult airway and have inspired individuals and institutions in other countries to develop guidelines. Examples are the Canadian Airway Focus Group (1998),

France (1996), SIAARTI Task Force (Italy, 1998) and Difficult Airway Society (UK, 2004).

2.1.1 Airway Guidelines share one or more of the following recommendations:

- derived by evidence-based analysis of current literature and consensus opinion;
- assist the anaesthetist in making decisions about difficult airway management;
- include formation of specific strategies (plans) for management of difficult airway;
- emphasize provision of oxygen to the patient at all times;
- emphasize avoidance of multiple attempts using the same airway technique;
- emphasize using alternative techniques to direct laryngoscopy;
- are usually summarized in algorithms;
- emphasize that training programmes should ensure that anaesthetists are trained in the use of airway techniques recommended in their algorithms.

2.1.2 Impact of guidelines on practice and training

It is tempting to suggest that by following the recommendations of difficult airway algorithms, anaesthetists would be able to manage each scenario successfully and that morbidity and/or mortality would be a thing of the past. The introduction of guidelines has certainly helped anaesthetists to plan and think about managing difficult airway scenarios in a structured way. The algorithms are not intended to be used as wall charts that could be accessed when problems occur but are designed as a tool to aid the anaesthetists' decision making skills. The guidelines form the basis of structured training in difficult airway management. Trainers can focus on these principles and teach sound principles of airway management to trainees. The Difficult Airway Society (DAS) algorithm recommends specific techniques for the unanticipated difficult intubation scenario in an adult non-obstetric patient. This is in the hope that these techniques would become 'core skills' that every anaesthetist should be able to perform. More importantly it would form the basis of training at workshops and/or on patients. Trainers can also use the recommendations in the guidelines as a 'lever' to purchase new equipment and overall create a 'difficult airway' friendly department. This in turn allows the individual anaesthetist to plan and execute a 'safe' airway management plan (see below).

2.2 Understanding difficult airway management

The principles of airway difficulties and their management are best understood by considering 'airway scenarios' and the following categorizations have been used in this book (Box 2.1). It must be understood that this is for discussion purposes only and in practice several of these scenarios may manifest in a

> **Box 2.1 Airway scenarios**
>
> **Anticipated Difficult Airway – 2.2.1**
> No upper airway obstruction – 2.2.1.1
> Clinical upper airway obstruction – 2.2.1.2
> **Unanticipated Difficult Intubation – 2.2.2**
> Can't intubate, can ventilate – 2.2.2.1
> During routine induction – 2.2.2.2
> During rapid sequence induction – 2.2.2.3
> **Can't Intubate, Can't Ventilate scenario – 2.2.3**
> **Special situations – 2.2.4**
> Patient centred – e.g. paediatric, obstetric, obesity – 2.2.4.1
> Environment centred – e.g. obstetric, major trauma – 2.2.4.2

single patient. Also some patient groups such as paediatrics, obstetrics, trauma and others present different challenges in differing environments but the fundamental principles remain the same and the scheme can also be used to facilitate safe airway management of these patients.

2.2.1 **Anticipated Difficult Airway**

2.2.1.1 *No upper airway obstruction*

The patient with anticipated difficulties whose airway cannot be readily managed using conventional airway techniques, e.g. direct laryngoscopy. This includes patients with anatomical or pathological problems who have little or no airway problems in their daily lives and when awake, but will do so if anaesthesia is induced injudiciously.

Management: Discussed in Chapter 5.

Gold standard: Awake Fibreoptic Intubation (AFI).

2.2.1.2 *With clinical upper airway obstruction*

The patient with upper airway compromise who, if left untreated, is at imminent risk of hypoxia and all its consequences

Management: Discussed in Chapter 6.

Gold standard: Individualized patient management depending on site, severity and progress of upper airway obstruction. Experience of the anaesthetist is crucial to management.

2.2.2 **Unanticipated difficult intubation**

The patient in whom airway difficulties occur despite a 'normal' pre operative assessment.

2.2.2.1 *Can't intubate, can ventilate*

In this scenario it is still possible to provide ventilation/oxygenation to the patient's lungs.

2.2.2.2 *During routine induction*

In this scenario there is no risk of aspiration of gastric contents and a non depolarizing relaxant has usually been used.

13

2.2.2.3 *During rapid sequence induction*

In this scenario there is risk of aspiration and suxamethonium has been used
Management: Discussed in Chapter 8.
Gold standard: DAS guideline techniques.

2.2.3 **Can't intubate, can't ventilate**

The patient in whom airway difficulties include the inability to secure tracheal
intubation but also the inability to provide oxygenation to the patient's lungs.
Management: Discussed in Chapter 9.
Gold standard: DAS guideline techniques.

2.2.4 **Special situations**

2.2.4.1 *Patient centred – e.g. paediatric, obstetric, obesity*

2.2.4.2 *Environment centred – e.g. obstetric, major trauma*

These patients may present with any of the scenarios (2.2.2.1 to 2.2.2.3) above
but their airway management poses 'special' challenges
Management: Discussed in Chapters 10 and 11.

2.2.5 **How should an anaesthetist approach difficult airway management?**

Managing a difficult airway is very often viewed with trepidation by many
anaesthetists. The knowledge that mismanagement may result in patient harm
including hypoxia, brain damage and death coupled with the need to follow the
recommendations of several guidelines is surely a daunting task. This is
compounded by the fact that since the incidence of failed ventilation/intubation
is very low anaesthetists may not have the experience of performing some of
the recommended techniques on a daily basis. It is also impossible for the
guidelines to cover all the possible scenarios and recommend specific
techniques for each of them.

The **5 'P's** scheme is a simple and practical way of managing each of the
difficult airway scenarios mentioned above. It is obvious that not all 'P's are
applicable to all the scenarios but their understanding allows the anaesthetist to
be better prepared. More importantly this scheme is a simplified way to take
into considerations all the principles and recommendations of airway guidelines.

In clinical practice the 'P's go hand in hand and are discussed here separately
for better understanding. It is vital that anaesthetists practice this scheme at
every opportunity, even when managing normal airways, so that the routine
not only allows them to safely manage the anticipated difficult airway scenarios
but also be prepared for the unanticipated difficulty.

2.2.5.1 *Preoperative airway assessment*

Routine airway assessment should include history, review of the patient's notes
especially the anaesthetic charts and performing bedside tests on every patient.
Often a potentially difficult airway is obvious by just 'eye-balling' the patient, for
example, severe restriction of mouth opening in a patient with previous oral

> **Box 2.2 The 5 'P's**
>
> 1. **Preoperative airway assessment**
> 2. **Planning**
> 3. **Procedures (techniques used to execute the plan)**
> 4. **Post procedure (extubation and follow up)**
> 5. **Publicity (telling others)**

cancer surgery and radiotherapy does not require further bedside tests to determine that intubation with direct laryngoscopy would be difficult. In less obvious cases bedside tests are recommended. The usefulness and limitations of bedside tests are discussed in Chapter 4.

Further categorization would include presence of clinical upper airway obstruction or not. The pre operative airway assessment of a patient with clinical upper airway obstruction is vital in determining the site, extent and progression of the obstruction and is discussed in Chapter 6.

The pre operative assessment allows the anaesthetist to categorize the patient into whether they are 'anticipated' to be difficult to intubate (with the intended intubation technique) and/or oxygenate (with the intended technique).

Most importantly, preoperative assessment and its findings allow the anaesthetist to 'think' difficult and hence make appropriate plans, as described below.

2.2.5.2 *Planning*

A well thought out and properly executed airway management plan is likely to result in a safe outcome. Planning not only includes decisions about the use of a specific airway technique or equipment but more importantly communicating these decisions to the surgeon, anaesthetic assistant and most important, to the patient.

2.2.5.2.1 *Plan A or primary plan*

This is the plan which has the best chance of success and which is safe for the nature of the airway difficulty identified at pre operative assessment. It is vital that the anaesthetist is experienced and familiar with the technique that is planned and that the patient consents to the technique. In the above example of the patient with restricted mouth opening, an awake intubation using a flexible fibreoptic scope would be an appropriate plan A. However, if the patient is a child or has learning difficulties, then an appropriate plan would be a suitable technique under general anaesthesia.

2.2.5.2.2 *Plan B or Back Up plan*

There should always be at least one back plan worked out in advance (plan B). Often the back up plan may include use of a piece of equipment not generally available or help from a colleague or even the surgeon. For this reason the back up plan should be thought out *before* the procedure, communicated to the appropriate personnel and arrangements made for the equipment/personnel to be available if needed. In the above example the anaesthetist may wish to consider either a technique under general anaesthesia or a surgical airway as a Plan B. This plan should be explained to the patient well in advance. The 'team' – surgeon, scrub staff, anaesthetic assistant – should be informed and necessary equipment should be in place.

2.2.5.3 *Procedures (techniques used to execute the plan)*

This 'P' is the step of executing the plan and includes the actual performance of the planned technique(s) to secure the airway. The incidence of difficult airway scenarios is small and not surprisingly there is lack of good, randomized, controlled trials of the use of equipment or techniques in patients who are truly difficult. For this reason it is difficult to give precise evidence based recommendations for each scenario.

Basic techniques such as face mask ventilation, LMA insertion/ventilation and an *optimum* technique of performing direct laryngoscopy are of paramount importance and all anaesthetists should aim to be experienced in their use. However, these would not allow one to safely secure the airway in some difficult airway scenarios and for this reason it is important to master some 'alternative' or 'advanced' techniques. The guidance on the use of these alternative techniques can be obtained from the various airway algorithms. The DAS algorithm in the UK deals with management of the unanticipated difficult intubation and also recommends specific techniques for each of the plans. The recognized (anticipated) part of the ASA algorithm recommend securing the airway while the patient is 'awake' – a safe and sensible approach. I find that combining the 'anticipated' part of the ASA algorithm and the DAS algorithm (for unanticipated difficulties) would cover *most* of the scenarios encountered in clinical practice (Figure 2.1). This approach also allows one to focus on mastering a small number of alternative (advanced) techniques. A list of basic and some of these advanced techniques is shown in Box 2.3. This list is by no means exhaustive. New airway equipment and techniques are being introduced at a frightening pace. Some of these are discussed in Chapter 13. It is very important that anaesthetists wishing to use any of these techniques in the difficult airway scenario first get the necessary experience in patients with normal airways.

2.2.5.4 *Post procedure (Extubation and follow up)*

Extubation can be more hazardous than intubation and needs to be carefully planned. Planning should include decisions about how extubation would be facilitated (either awake or in the anaesthetized patient) and more importantly how the patient would be re intubated should the need arise in the recovery phase. The focus should be on maintaining oxygenation of the patient at all times. Extubation and re intubation of the difficult airway are discussed in Chapter 12.

A follow up interview with the patient is mandatory. Where management has gone according to plan, it allows the anaesthetist to get valuable feedback from the patient and allows him/her to improve techniques. Where complications have occurred, especially trauma, it is vital to examine the patient, document the injuries, and actively seek signs of pharyngolaryngeal perforation. These may present late and can be life threatening.

Box 2.3 List of procedures to implement airway management plans
• Face Mask Ventilation
• LMA insertion/ventilation
• *Optimized* attempt at direct laryngoscopy
• Mastering at least two alternative direct laryngoscopes, e.g. McCoy, Straight Blade
• Mastering at least one indirect laryngoscope, e.g. Airtraq, Glidescope, McGrath
• Fibreoptic intubation (oral and nasal)
• Fibreoptic assisted intubation through LMA
• Blind/Fibreoptic intubation through ILMA
• Awake fibreoptic intubation
• Cannula cricothyroidotomy and jet ventilation

2.2.5.5 *Publicity (telling others)*

The anaesthetist has a duty of care to inform the patient of any airway problems he/she had encountered in their management. Details of the airway management and problems encountered and their solutions should be explicit. This detailed information would be very useful for the anaesthetist managing that patient in the future Communication should also be made with the surgeon and the patients GP. Ideally a national database of such patients would be useful but one does not exist in the UK. The author uses the 'Airway Alert' scheme described Dr David Ball in Dumphries. The form is available to download from the DAS website (www.das.uk.com).

2.3 10 golden rules of safe (difficult) airway management

1. Develop you *own* scheme of pre operative airway assessment and always use it.
2. Always work out airway management plans (strategies) in *advance.*
3. Work out at least one *back up* plan and get things ready.
4. Ensure that your *basic* airway skills are impeccable.
5. Master a few alternative *advanced* airway skills.
6. Keep your skills up to date by using them *regularly.*
7. Audit your practice, make changes and learn *new* skills.
8. Make it your duty to *teach* these skills to others.
9. Remember to plan extubation as meticulously as intubation.
10. Always prioritize *oxygenation* over everything else!!!

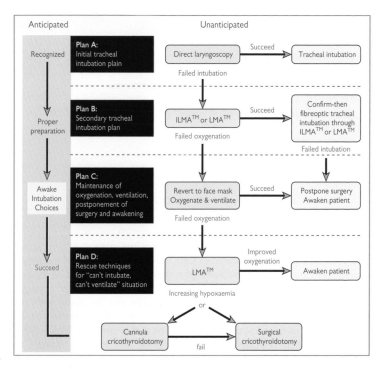

Figure 2.1 Combining the ASA algorithm for the 'anticipated' (recognized) and the DAS algorithm for unanticipated difficulties. This approach covers most scenarios and focuses on mastering a small number of alternative techniques.

Further reading

Airway alert form http://www.das.uk.com/guidelines/airwayalert.html.

American Society of Anaesthetists Task Force on Management of Difficult Airway. Practice Guidelines for Management of the Difficult Airway. An Updated Report. Anesthesiology 2003; **98**:1269–77. http://www.asahq.org/publicationsAndServices/DifficultAirway.pdf.

Ball DR, Jefferson P. Airway management training for all. *Anaesthesia*; 2003 **58**: 185–6.

Barron FA, Ball DR, Jefferson P, Norrie J. 'Airway Alerts'. How UK anaesthetists organise, document and communicate difficult airway management. Anaesthesia; **58**: 73–7.

Crosby ET, Cooper RM, Douglas MJ et al. The unanticipated difficult airway with recommendations for management. Canadian Journal of Anaesthesia 1998; **45**: 757–76.

Henderson JJ, Popat MT, Latto IP, Pearce AC: Difficult Airway Society guidelines for management of the unanticipated difficult intubation. *Anaesthesia* 2004; **59**: 675–94.

http://www.das.uk.com/guidelines/guidelineshome.html.

http://anestit.unipa.it/siaarti/Intubazing.htm.

Italian Society of Anaesthesiology Analgesia Reanimation and Intensive Care. SIAARTI (siaarti societa' italiana di anestesia analgesia rianimazione e terapia intensiva) guidelines for difficult intubation and for difficult airway management *Minerva Anestesiologica* 1998; **64**: 361–71.

Popat M. The Airway. *Anaesthesia* 2003; **58**: 1166–1171.

Chapter 3

Basic anatomical, physiological and pharmacological principles of difficult airway management

Jaideep J. Pandit

Key points
• Understanding of 'normal' upper airway anatomy is essential in safe execution of airway management procedures
• Variants of upper airway anatomy due to whatever cause may make airway management difficult
• Understanding the pathophysiology of airway compromise and its consequences is paramount in providing safe airway management.
• Understanding pharmacology of agents used for airway procedures aids in their success.

3.1 Upper airway anatomy

The human airway has two openings: the nose and the mouth. The floor of the nose is the roof of the mouth. Separated by the palate (which has two components; an anterior hard palate and a posterior soft palate), these two passages join posteriorly in the pharynx, the nose leading to the nasopharynx and the mouth to the oropharynx.

3.1.1 The nose

The nasal septum divides the nasal cavity into two fossae or passages, which open anteriorly at the nares and posteriorly into the nasopharynx at the choanae. The fossae are lined by mucus membrane and within its lateral wall

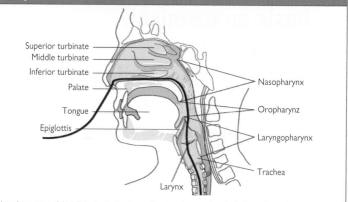

Figure 3.1 Simplified line diagram showing main structures of the upper airway

Superior turbinate
Middle turbinate
Inferior turbinate
Palate
Tongue
Epiglottis

Nasopharynx
Oropharynx
Laryngopharynx
Trachea
Larynx

Note the position of the inferior turbinate; airway adjuncts such as nasal tracheal tube or fibreoptic scope are passed directly backwards perpendicular to the plane of the face and directed below the inferior turbinate. Note also that the 'angle' of passage with a nasal airway adjunct is less acute than with an oral one. Note that although the soft palate and tongue are shown as if some distance apart, in reality they are often apposed and form a 'barrier' to successful oral fibreoptic-assisted intubation. Note that the epiglottis is positioned to protect the laryngeal inlet: in some patients a large or floppy epiglottis is a cause of a difficult intubation.

are found three irregular ridges projecting medially: the superior, middle and inferior turbinates (conchae). The space beneath each turbinate is called a meatus into which open the paranasal sinuses. It should be noted that the usual pathway for insertion of airway adjuncts (tubes, airways, fibreoptic scope) is *below* the inferior turbinate. The axis of the nasal cavity is perpendicular to the face and so these adjuncts should be inserted directly backwards.

3.1.2 **The mouth**

The oral cavity is bound by the alveolus and the teeth in the front and laterally, the floor of the mouth is largely occupied by the anterior two thirds of the tongue (the posterior one third is in the oropharynx) and the roof is formed by the hard and soft palate. The external muscles of the tongue connect it to the various structures, e.g. the genioglossus muscle which attaches the tongue to the mandible. Their weakness or paralysis due to anaesthesia, trauma or infection may lead to backward displacement of the tongue and airway obstruction.

3.1.3 **The pharynx**

The pharynx is a U-shaped fibromuscular structure that connects the nasal and oral cavities to the larynx and the oesophagus. Sub-divided into the nasopharynx, oropharynx, and hypopharynx it extends from the base of the skull to the inferior border of the cricoid cartilage anteriorly (at the entrance of the oesophagus) and the inferior border of the C6 vertebra posteriorly. The wall of the pharynx is composed of two layers of pharyngeal muscles (external circular and internal longitudinal layer), which elevate the larynx and pharynx during swallowing and speaking.

The nasopharynx lies directly behind the nasal cavity and may have enlarged lymphoid or adenoid tonsil tissues along its roof and lateral walls, making nasotracheal intubation difficult.

The oropharynx begins where the nasopharynx ends at the soft palate superiorly and extends inferiorly to the tip of the epiglottis. The lateral walls contain the paired tonsillar fossae which may contain enlarged palatine tonsils making direct laryngosocpy difficult. Hypertrophy of the lingual tonsil (above the epiglottis) is a known cause of unanticipated difficult laryngoscopy with the Macintosh blade (Chapter 8). The glossopharyngel nerve can be blocked at the base of glossopalatal fold (Chapter 7). This block is useful for abolishing the gag reflex.

The hypopharynx (or laryngopharynx) extends from the upper border of the epiglottis to the lower border of the cricoid cartilage (between the 4th and 6th cervical vertebra). It is continuous above with the oropharynx and below with both the oesophagus and laryngeal inlet.

The laryngeal inlet lies anteriorly in the hypophayrnx and is defined by the epiglottis, the aryepiglottic folds, the arytenoid cartilages and the posterior commisure. The epiglottis is a spoon shaped plate of elastic cartilage that lies behind the tongue (Figure 3.2). It prevents aspiration by covering the glottis – the opening of the larynx – during swallowing. On each side are the pyriform fossae which divert food boluses laterally and away from the larynx in transit to the oesophagus. The paired lateral glossoepiglottic folds and the single median fold bound two spaces called the epiglottic vallecula and attach the tongue to the epiglottis. The valleculae are where a curved laryngoscope blade is inserted in order to lift the epiglottis and visualize the glottis. Posteriorly the bucco-pharyngeal and prevertebral fascia can be the site of pharyngeal tears during traumatic laryngoscopy.

3.1.4 **The larynx**

The larynx is a cartilaginous skeleton held together by ligaments and muscles and serves as a valve to prevent passage of food/drink into the lungs during swallowing (closed valve), and also contains the vocal cords which regulate speech (partially closed valve) and an open valve in respiration. The nine cartilages of the larynx are: thyroid, cricoid, epiglottis, and (in pairs) the arytenoid, corniculate and cuneiform. All the intrinsic muscles of the larynx adduct (i.e. close) the vocal cords, except the posterior crico-arytenoid muscles, innervated by the recurrent laryngeal nerve. Hence damage to this nerve in laryngeal, thoracic or neck surgery can cause partial or complete airway obstruction due to loss of vocal cord abduction.

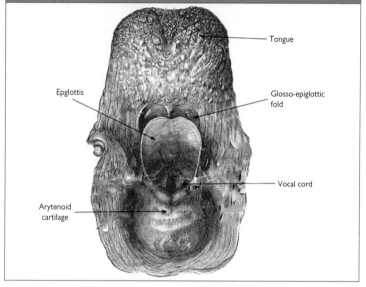

Figure 3.2 **Diagrammatic view of the larynx, as it appears with tracheal intubation using a Macintosh laryngoscope**

Tongue

Epglottis

Glosso-epiglottic fold

Vocal cord

Arytenoid cartilage

The cricoid cartilage is of clinical relevance as the site of exertion of cricoid pressure during a rapid sequence induction of anaesthesia. This action compresses the oesophagus posteriorly and thus helps prevent regurgitation of material from the stomach into the pharynx (and hence into the lungs). However, improperly applied force on the cricoid carltilage can also make the laryngeal view during laryngoscopy more difficult. The cricothyroid membrane is the site for a surgical cricothyroidotomy (Chapter 9). The advantage of this site is that the membrane is thin, with ready access to the airway, and relatively avascular, away from cardinal structures in the neck (Figure 3.3).

This chapter will not contain a detailed description of the trachea, except to state that it is about 9–15 cm in length in the adult and bifurcates into the right and left main bronchi at the carina (level of the sternal angle, ~T4 vertebral level). The trachea is the site for a more formal surgical tracheostomy (Figure 3.3).

3.2 **The anatomy of a 'difficult airway'**

The above description applies to the 'normal' airway anatomy; difficulties in mask ventilation and/or tracheal intubation generally arise due to altered anatomy resulting from normal variations or due to pathology, surgery, or radiotherapy. Some examples are given below but the details are covered in the relevant chapters.

Figure 3.3 Surface anatomy (diagrammatic) of the larynx

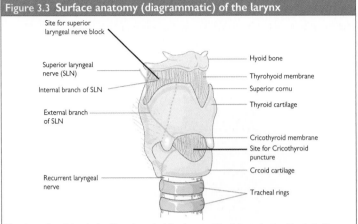

Site for superior
laryngeal nerve block

Superior laryngeal
nerve (SLN)

Internal branch of SLN

External branch
of SLN

Recurrent laryngeal
nerve

Hyoid bone

Thyrohyoid membrane

Superior cornu

Thyroid cartilage

Cricothyroid membrane

Site for Cricothyroid
puncture

Crcoid cartilage

Tracheal rings

Note the position of the cricothyroid membrane (and site of puncture) in relation to the thyroid and cricoid cartilages. Superiorly is the hyoid bone with its greater cornu as the spot where the superior laryngeal nerve may be blocked by injection (see Chapter 7).

3.2.1 Difficult mask ventilation

It may be difficult to hold a facemask on a patient's face securely and hand-ventilate the lungs because of: presence of beard; dentures (that cause poor facemask seal on a 'floppy' face, and leak of oxygen); altered facial anatomy (e.g. extensive facial injury, external metal fixator devices; ankylosis of tempero-mandibular joints); obesity; a large tongue (e.g. in Down's syndrome) or tumours of the oral cavity (see Chapter 4).

3.2.2 Difficult laryngoscopy

Standard laryngoscopy with a Macintosh blade involves placing its tip in the vallecula and then lifting the epiglottis thus exposing the vocal cords to a direct line of view (Figure 3.4). Thus any abnormality that prevents this sequence of events will predispose to difficulty in viewing the vocal cords and hence intubation. Any of the factors that make mask ventilation difficult might also make intubation difficult. The management of the anticipated and unanticipated difficult intubation is discussed in Chapters 5 and 8.

These anatomical considerations lead to an important – and logical – conclusion. Almost all patients with even extreme forms of the conditions listed above have a normal ability to breathe when awake and in their daily lives. It is only when anaesthesia is induced that airway obstruction becomes problematic, and that manoeuvres involving the laryngoscope are restricted. The logical conclusion is that all risks to these patients arise from induction of anaesthesia. Therefore, it seems further logical to secure the airway of those patients identified to be potentially difficult when these patients are awake (or sedated) and before induction of anaesthesia (Chapter 5).

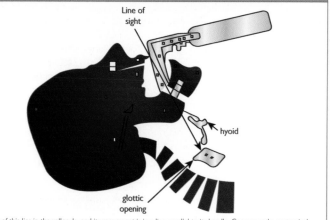

Figure 3.4 Diagram of conventional tracheal intubation with Macintosh laryngoscope

Line of sight

hyoid

glottic opening

The tip of this lies in the vallecula, and its movement is in a line parallel to its handle. Consequently, anatomical structures are moved anteriorly and the larynx is brought into the 'line of sight'.

Acute airway compromise does, however, happen due to airway obstruction (Chapter 6). It is therefore important to understand the pathophysiology of the compromised obstructed airway and ensuing hypoxia and hypoventilation.

3.2.3 Pathophysiology of upper airway obstruction

As implied above, collapse of any of the upper airway tissues will obstruct the free movement of air in and out of the lungs. This of course happens during normal induction of anaesthesia, but is also exacerbated by certain pathologies such as acute epiglottitis or tumours of the upper airway. The conventional airway manoeuvres practiced by anaesthetists (e.g. head extension, chin lift, with or without a Guedel airway) to some extent mitigate the airway collapse but cannot guarantee free movement of air in all situations. In such a 'can't ventilate' scenario it is useful to consider some of the physiology that eventually leads to hypoxia.

The 'oxygen capacity' of the body is for all practical purposes contained in the haemoglobin and in the volume of air in the lungs (the functional residual capacity). There are ~5 litres of blood in a normal adult and each litre carries ~200ml O_2 bound to haemoglobin (thus totalling ~1 litre of O_2). The functional residual capacity of the lungs in an adult is ~3 L, of which just 20% is oxygen (~600 ml), making a total of 1.6 L of O_2 available for metabolism. Since the basal O_2 consumption is ~250 ml/min, this means that if ventilation ceases, there is a ~6 min supply before all the O_2 in the body is consumed (and much shorter before arterial hypoxaemia as detectable by a pulse oximeter occurs). Clearly this is not very long and indeed this time may be shortened if, for example, an obstructed patient is struggling for breath or tachycardic with anxiety (and thus increasing their O_2 consumption). If by good chance the patient has been effectively preoxygenated, this will greatly increase the time available before the body stores are depleted. Preoxygenation will not change much the O_2 carried by the blood, but it will mean that most of the 3L of lung capacity is oxygen, thus extending the time available to ~16 min (Figure 3.5).

Even a very small degree of ventilation of the lungs is useful in this situation (e.g. gas flow even via a 'pinhole' conduit in the obstructed tissues). Since the body is consuming O_2 at 250 ml/min, this can be conceived as creating a partial pressure gradient in favour of oxygen flow towards the lungs – O_2 will flow through even the smallest aperture, even if visible movement of the chest with manual ventilation appears impossible, and this will further extend the time available to a rescuer. Thus even in the 'can't ventilate' scenario, it is worthwhile maintaining a tight facemask seal with an O_2 suppy or via a laryngeal mask airway, in case a subclinical conduit for O_2 flow exists within the obstruction.

The body excretes CO_2 also at a rate of ~250 ml/min. However, the body's capacity to store CO_2 is very large indeed so very little of this CO_2 produced by metabolism is translated into a rise in arterial partial pressure of CO_2. Thus PCO_2 only rises at a rate of ~0.5 kPa/min during an obstructed or apnoeic airway. While this certainly contributes to a degree of acidosis, even quite high levels of PCO_2 (e.g., 15-20 kPa) are not fatal so there is at least 20–30 min available

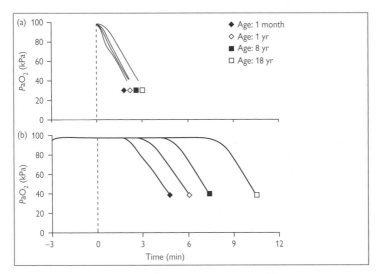

Figure 3.5 Top panel A: decline in artrerial PO_2 with time without preoxygenation in different age groups. Bottom panel C: decline after preoxygenation; note the dramatic effect in adults, and note also the improved (but still more rapid) decline in children.

Reproduced from Hardman JG and Wills JS, The development of hypoxaemia during apnoea in children: a computational modeling investigation, *British Journal of Anaesthesia* (2006), **97**(4): 564–70, with permission of Oxford University Press.

before CO_2 accumulation is a significant problem for survival. Note also that, as for oxygen, even a pinhole conduit will assist flow of CO_2 out of the lungs as it facilitates flow of O_2 into the lungs.

3.3 Pharmacology relevant to airway management

Techniques such as awake intubation are accomplished using judicious sedation and local anaesthesia of the upper airway. Inhalational induction of anaesthesia is also a technique used where awake intubation is not feasible. This section of the chapter deals with the pharmacology of the drugs used for these techniques:

- drugs used for conscious sedation;
- drugs used for local anaesthesia of the upper airway;
- agents used for inhalational anaesthesia.

3.3.1 Drugs used for conscious sedation

3.3.1.1 *Benzodiazepines*

Benzodiazepines are good sedative, anxiolytic and amnesic drugs. They have no analgesic action.

3.3.1.2 *Midazolam*

This water soluble benzodiazepine produces no pain on intravenous injection. It has a quick onset and short duration of action. Hypotension and respiratory depression are minimal when midazolam is given in small doses but may occur with large doses and when the drug is combined with opioids, in the elderly and patients with respiratory disease. Midazolam is contraindicated in patients with human immune deficiency disorders who are on protease inhibitors which may significantly alter the CNS effects of midazolam due to alteration of cytochrome P 450 activity resulting in increased plasma concentrations. The effects of midazolam can be quickly reversed with a specific antagonist; flumazenil should over dosage cause respiratory depression or airway obstruction. The initial dose of flumazenil is 0.2 mg and this can be repeated.

3.3.2 Opioids

When given alone, opioids produce sedation but no anxiolysis or amnesia. They are powerful analgesics and suppress the cough reflex.

3.3.2.1 *Fentanyl*

Fentanyl is a phenylpiperidine derivative and is 100 times more potent than morphine. It has a quick onset and short duration of action due to redistribution in inactive tissues such as fat and muscle. Unlike morphine, fentanyl does not produce histamine release, thus reducing the risk of hypotension. Chest tightness may occur with rapid injection. It may cause respiratory depression and drowsiness especially when combined with midazolam.

3.3.2.2 *Alfentanil*

Alfentanil is 10 times weaker than fentanyl but has a slightly faster onset of action. It may be diluted to 100 μg/ml and given as boluses of one to two ml at a time.

3.3.2.3 *Remifentanil*

Remifentanil may have some advantages over the fentanyl congeners in providing the opioid component of sedation and analgesia for CS. Because of the ester structure, it is susceptible to ester hydrolysis resulting in rapid metabolism. It effects dissipate very quickly after an infusion is stopped. It has a very rapid onset rendering titration of the infusion precisely controllable. Changes in the administration rate are quickly reflected in the level of drug effect. If an opioid effect is desirable then it can be quickly achieved with an increase in infusion rate. If toxic effects such as decreased respiratory rate or apnoea result, then stopping the infusion will quickly reverse these effects. Infusion rates of between 0.05 and 0.175 μg/kg/minute have been used for awake fibreoptic intubation.

3.3.3 **Naloxone**

Naloxone is a specific mu receptor antagonist. It reverses not only the respiratory depression but also the analgesic effects of opioids. It may also cause CNS excitation. One way to administer naloxone is to dilute it 40 μg/ml (400 μg in 10 ml normal saline) and give one to two ml at a time, titrating the dose to effect.

3.3.4 **Propofol**

Propofol is a phenol derivative that has been used as an anaesthetic since 1989. The painful intravenous injection can be prevented by prior injection of a small dose of lidocaine. Its advantages are a quick onset of action and rapid recovery due to redistribution from the central to the peripheral compartment. Propofol weakens the upper airway reflexes and is particularly suited to local anaesthetic techniques involving airway manipulation. It is easy to administer propofol with simple infusion pumps. The dose is variable and can be titrated between 0.5–2 mg/kg/hr. A simple and effective way of administering propofol by infusion is to give it on a mg/min basis regardless of patient weight and age, the usual dose being 1–2 mg/min. Target controlled infusion (TCI) of propofol is also commonly used in anaesthesia. TCI propofol in a dosage range of 0.8–1.2 μg/ml has been used for CS during awake fibreoptic intubation. The pump is simple and titration of propofol is easy in maintaining the desired sedation level and cardio respiratory stability. Propofol does not provide amnesia and it may be necessary to administer a small dose of midazolam (0.5–1mg) before commencing propofol infusion to ensure amnesia. Overdose with propofol may cause unconsciousness, respiratory depression and hypotension. There is no specific antidote available for reversing these effects.

Practical techniques of conscious sedation for awake fibreoptic intubation are discussed in Chapter 7.

3.4 **Drugs used for local anaesthesia of upper airway**

3.4.1 **Local anaesthetics**

Local anaesthetics act by preventing depolarization of the nerve membranes that follows influx of sodium. Local anaesthetics are available as water soluble acidic salts and when injected or topically applied, they are buffered in the tissues releasing the free base. The free base is lipid soluble and penetrates the nerve tissue producing anaesthesia. The release of the free base is delayed and the action of local anaesthetic is slow when the pH and buffering capacity of the tissues is lowered as in infection. Topical local anaesthetics are less effective than injection techniques because of the low buffering capacity of the mucous membranes. A higher concentration of local anaesthetic is therefore required for topical anaesthesia. In the respiratory tract, the absorption of local anaesthetic is more rapid from the tracheobronchial tree, than from the pharynx. Vasoconstrictors added to local anaesthetics for topical anaesthesia neither delay absorption nor prolong the duration of the action. Systemic effects of local anaesthetics are related to their plasma concentration. This depends on a variety of factors such as the total dose used, rate of absorption, distribution and metabolism. Metabolism is slow in patients with hepatic disease.

3.4.1.1 *Cocaine*

Cocaine is a natural alkaloid obtained from the leaves of Erythroxylon Coca. It is the only local anaesthetic with vasoconstrictor properties. The vasoconstrictor properties are due to interference with re uptake of circulating catecholamine by the adrenergic nerve endings, the delay increasing catecholamine blood levels and producing vasoconstriction. Cocaine is an ester local anaesthetic, readily absorbed from the respiratory mucosa and slowly metabolised by pseudocholinesterase. Cocaine is available as 5% and 10% solution but it is a controlled drug. The 5% solution takes about 3–5 minutes to act, maximum plasma levels are reached in 60 minutes and metabolism takes 5–6 hours. The 10% solution has a faster onset but may cause toxicity and should not be used. Signs of systemic toxicity include hypertension, tachycardia and cardiac arrhythmia. Body temperature may rise. The drug has powerful cortical stimulating action and may cause excitement, euphoria and increase in mental alertness. Cocaine in a dose of 2 mg/kg has been shown to cause coronary artery vasoconstriction with a reduction in coronary blood flow and increased myocardial oxygen demands. Cocaine should be used with caution in patients with hypertension, coronary artery disease, pre eclampsia and with pseudocholinesterase deficiency. The maximum recommended dose of cocaine for topical anaesthesia of the nasal cavity is 1.5 mg/kg or 100 mg in a fit adult.

3.4.1.2 *Lidocaine*

Lidocaine is an amide local anaesthetic and is the most common drug used for local anaesthesia of the respiratory tract. It is a vasodilator and has bitter taste. Many different topical preparations of lidocaine are available such as aqueous 1%, 2% and 4% or viscous (gel) 2%, ointment 5%, 10% metered spray (10 mg per spray). The 4% solution is commonly used for topical anaesthesia of the upper airway and its action lasts for 15–20 minutes. The 2% solution is less effective and takes longer.

The rate of absorption of lidocaine depends on the surface area of the respiratory tract, the method of topical anaesthesia and whether the patient is breathing spontaneously or is anaesthetised and ventilated. Absorption of lidocaine is slower in the upper respiratory tract (oropharynx, nasopharynx, and larynx) than the lower respiratory tract (bronchi, alveoli) because of its smaller surface area. A fraction of the lidocaine sprayed onto the oropharynx is removed during suctioning and some of it may be swallowed. About 70% of the swallowed lidocaine is metabolised in the liver at first pass. The plasma concentration of lidocaine is therefore lower with upper respiratory tract application than during lower respiratory tract application. Once in the plasma, lidocaine is metabolized by the hepatic microsomal system. Lower doses of lidocaine should be used in patients with hepatic disease and low cardiac output states. In the conscious patient, toxic symptoms may appear with plasma levels of about 5 μg/ml. The maximum recommended dose of lidocaine for topical application to the respiratory tract is 200 mg in an adult. In practice higher doses have been used without systemic toxicity and peak plasma levels below the toxic levels described.

3.4.2 **Vasoconstrictors**

The nasal mucosa is highly vascular and may bleed on instrumentation. Blood interferes with the fibreoptic view. It is therefore necessary to combine vasoconstriction when topical anaesthesia of the nasal mucosa is performed. Cocaine is both a local anaesthetic and vasoconstrictor but some anaesthetists routinely avoid its use for fear of toxicity. Its use is also contraindicated in certain conditions (see above). Other vasoconstrictors, usually mixed with lidocaine, may then be used to produce local anaesthesia and vasoconstriction.

3.4.2.1 *Xylometazoline 0.1%*

Xylometazoline is a sympathomimetic compound commonly used as a nasal decongestant in a spray form or as drops. It has been found to be as effective as cocaine in producing nasal vasoconstriction. For topical anaesthesia of the nasal cavity (unlicensed use), 5–10 drops (0.5 ml) are mixed with 4 ml of 4% lidocaine or 2% gel to produce satisfactory anaesthesia and vasoconstriction.

3.4.2.2 *Phenylephrine*

Phenylephrine is an alpha agonist and a powerful vasoconstrictor. For topical anaesthesia and vasoconstriction of the nasal cavity, 4ml of 4% lidocaine and

1 ml of 1% phenylephrine are mixed resulting in a mixture of 3.2% lidocaine and 0.2% phenylephrine. A commercial mixture is also available.

Methods of delivery of local anaesthetic and vasoconstrictors for awake intubation are discussed in Chapter 7.

3.4.3 Agents used for inhalation induction

3.4.3.1 Sevoflurane

Sevoflurane is a halogenated ether with relatively low blood-gas solubility which means that it has rapid onset of action (and rapid elimination). Since it is also non-irritant to the airway, it is particularly suitable for inhalational induction of anaesthesia. The broad principle of this technique is that, in cases where difficulty with the airway is expected, sevoflurane will enable anaesthesia to deepen so long as the patient breathes it in. If for any reason there is airway obstruction (ie, the airway is 'lost'), then uptake of sevoflurane will cease, the patient will awaken and thus become able again to maintain their own airway. Rapid recovery from sevoflurane anaesthesia – and hence rapid restoration of the ability to self-maintain the airway – is also an advantage in patients with difficult airways. Finally, respiratory control is preserved best with sevoflurane. At sub-anaesthetic doses (i.e., as during the revovery phase from anaesthesia) ventilatory responses to hypoxia and hypercapnia are maintained with sevoflurane (while with other volatile agents these are severly blunted) and clinically, a tachypnoea is often observed. Taken together, it therefore seems logical to use sevoflurane not only in the induction phase, but also in the maintenance of anaesthesia for patients with difficult airways (although the evidence base for this advice remains lacking).

Further reading

Boerner TF, Ramanathan S. Functional Anatomy of the Airway. In Benumof JL (ed) *Airway Management Principles and Practice*. Philadelphia, Mosby 1996, pp. 3–21.

Efthimiou J, Higenbottam T, Holt D, Cochrane GM. Plasma concentrationsof lidocaine during fibreoptic bronchoscopy. *Thorax* 1982; **37**: 68–71.

Hardman JG and Wills JS. The development of hypoxaemia during apnoea in children: a computational modelling investigation. *British Journal of Anaesthesia* 2005; **97**: 564–70.

Knolle E, Oehmke MJ, Gustorff B, Hellwagner K, Kress HG. Target controlled infusion of propofol for fibreoptic intubation. *Eur J Anaesthesiol* 2003; **20**: 565–9.

Pandit JJ. Volatile anesthetics and the hypoxic ventilatory response: effects, clinical implications, and future research. *Seminars in Anesthesia, Perioperative Medicine & Pain* 2007; **26**: 49–57.

Pandit JJ. Intravenous anaesthetic agents. *Anaesthesia & Intensive Care Medicine* 2008; **9**: 154–9.

Pandit JJ, Duncan T, Robbins PA. Total oxygen uptake with two maximal breathing techniques and the tidal volume technique: A physiologic study of preoxygenation. *Anesthesiology* 2003; **99**: 841–6.

Popat M. Practical Fibreoptic Intubation. Butterworth Heinemann, Oxford 2001.

Puchner W, Egger P, Puhringer F, *et al.* Evaluation of remifentanil as a single drug for awake fibreoptic intubation. *Acta Anaesthesiol Scand* 2002; **46**: 350–4.

Redden RJ. Anatomic airway considerations in anaesthesia. In Hagberg C (ed) *Handbook of Difficult Airway Management*, Philadelphia, Churchill Livingstone 2000, pp. 1–13.

Woodall NM, Harwood RJ, Barker GL, *et al.* Lidocaine toxicity in volunteer subjects undergoing awake fibreoptic intubation. *Anesth Analg* 2005; **101**: 606–15.

Chapter 4

Preoperative airway assessment

Chris Frerk and Kawshala Peiris

Key points

- If you only know one way to manage an airway, an airway assessment is of no value
- The statistical relevance of a test is different to the clinical relevance of a test
- False positive and false negative results are unavoidable
- Assessing the airway preoperatively will allow you to choose the most appropriate and safest management technique, prepare back-up plans, and organize any extra equipment and personnel that may be required
- If two out of three tests predict difficulty prepare for trouble.

There is a belief amongst some anaesthetists that preoperative airway assessment is not worthwhile and it has even been described as a useless ritual! This chapter will help you understand the value of preoperative airway assessment and how it can be applied usefully to reduce risk to patients.

4.1 The purpose of preoperative airway assessment

The purpose of preoperative airway assessment is to identify patients likely to be difficult to intubate, oxygenate or both. For more than 50 years anaesthetists have been trying to identify patients with difficult airways preoperatively to avoid having to manage them unexpectedly after induction of anaesthesia. Ideally it would be possible to correctly predict ease or difficulty with facemask ventilation, ventilation via a laryngeal mask (and other supraglottic airways) and with tracheal intubation (using various laryngoscopes). More than 20 tests have been described as predictors of difficult intubation (Box 4.1) and the number of statistical tests used to evaluate the effectiveness of predictors runs into double figures (Box 4.2).

Box 4.1 Airway assessment tests

- Mallampati test and Samsoon and Young's modification;
- Wilson score (a sum of scores from five variables);
- Thyromental distance;
- Sternomental distance;
- Ratio of height to thyromental distance;
- Upper lip bite test;
- Mandibular subluxation;
- Interdental distance;
- Bull neck;
- Neck circumference;
- Receding jaw;
- Buck teeth;
- Missing teeth;
- Sentinel teeth;
- Weight;
- The prayer sign;
- El-Ganzouri multivariate risk index (a score based on seven risk factors including previous difficulty);
- Head and neck movement;
- Goniometry;
- Radiological tests Atlanto axial gap and various angles;
- Exploratory direct laryngoscopy.

Box 4.2 Statistical tests that have been used to evaluate screening tests

- Sensitivity;
- Specificity;
- Positive predictive value;
- Negative predictive value;
- Positive and negative likelihood ratios;
- Positive and negative post test probabilities;
- Odds ratios;
- Relative risk;
- Accuracy;
- Precision;
- Areas under receiver operating characteristic (ROC) curves.

4.2 Limitations of predictive tests

The vast majority of the physical features and tests described have been aimed at predicting difficult laryngoscopy with a Macintosh laryngoscope. It is important to realize that these tests are not necessarily transferable to other methods of airway management, nor from one population to another with variations described between racial groups.

The tests that have been evaluated for use of the Macintosh laryngoscope principally aim to identify factors that make it difficult to align oral pharyngeal and tracheal axes and gain a direct line of sight to the larynx. When the Macintosh fails in these situations other devices may expose the larynx – the McCoy can sometimes lift the epiglottis when the Macintosh cannot, straight blades may be able to displace the tongue when the Macintosh cannot and most importantly for the future, video laryngoscopes can effectively 'see round corners' using either video or fibreoptic technology. There is very little information published relating to predictive tests for anything other than intubation with the Macintosh laryngoscope. A large study looking at difficulty with mask ventilation was published in 2006 and the first paper looking at risk factors for difficulty with a video laryngoscope (the Glidescope) was published in December 2007. Even the best preoperative predictor of difficulty (previous failure) only applies to the technique or instrument used on the previous occasion. There are well documented cases of confirmed grade 3 and 4 Macintosh intubation failures that have been easy grade 1 or 2 intubations with a different laryngoscope blade, and of failed facemask ventilation that has become possible simply with insertion of a nasopharyngeal airway.

Unless we are able to understand the information obtained from tests there is no value in performing them.

4.3 Understanding what the tests can tell us

The aim of a screening test is to identify people with a condition from within a population. We make an assumption that there are two distinct groups within the population that can be separated by the test. If this were the case a cut off point could be chosen for the test with all the difficult patients lying on one side and the rest of the population on the other (Figure 4.1).

When it comes to airway management there is significant overlap between the two groups but it is still important to choose a cut off point below which all patients are treated as difficult. There is no right or wrong cut off point, but choosing one does have an effect on the number of false positive and false negative results (Figure 4.2).

Neither A, B nor C in Figure 4.2 is intrinsically 'right'; it is up to each anaesthetist to determine whether they consider false alarms more of a problem than missed cases and to choose a cut off point based on that decision. To keep the test objective it is important to decide on the cut off point at which anaesthetic management will be changed, before the test is performed.

4.4 Statistical versus clinical evaluation

For research purposes tests need to be evaluated to attempt to determine their usefulness.

For a test such as interincisor gap each patient will have mouth opening measured in millimetres, giving a population spread, along with a record of whether

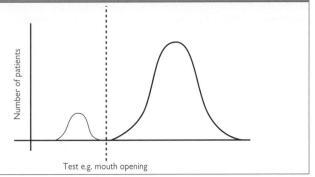

Figure 4.1 Ideal Screening Test. Patients with the condition being tested for are represented by the small curve (left) and the normal population by the larger curve (right)

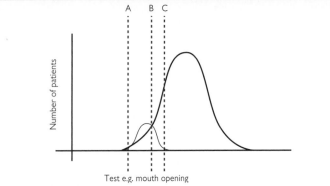

Figure 4.2 Example of Difficult Airway Screening Test with significant overlap

A gives no false alarms but the number of difficult cases picked up is low.

B is a pragmatic cut off point for the test, picking up a significant proportion of the difficult cases and keeping false alarms to a minimum.

C all difficult cases are detected but there are a significant number of false alarms.

airway management was easy or difficult. Statistical tests can be applied to every distance to determine how likely each result is to indicate difficulty with the airway.

The clinician at the bedside however only wants a yes/no answer to the question 'Is the patient likely to be difficult?' So when it comes to bedside testing a single cut off point is needed to make the decision. Again it is important to stress that there is no right or wrong cut off point. One anaesthetist may choose an interincisor distance of 2mm as a cut off point – he or she will have no false positive results. Another may choose 20 mm and will therefore be getting the fibrescope out more often, sometimes unnecessarily.

Similarly the Mallampati test has three grades, the Samsoon & Young modification of Mallampati has four grades each of which could be analysed statistically. At the bedside the test needs only two grades (with a single cut off point – easy or difficult). The same is true of any bedside screening test.

4.5 Why anaesthetists believe the tests don't work

Serious difficulty with airway management is uncommon so any reduction in incidence is unlikely to be noticed without careful audit. The advantages of testing are therefore difficult for the individual anaesthetist to appreciate in their normal practice. However, every false result encountered in day to day anaesthesia serves to reinforce the idea that the test is useless. If a test predicts that a case will be difficult, then after intubation with a fibrescope or by a consultant who is called in specially to assist, Macintosh laryngoscopy turns out to be straightforward – the belief that testing is useless is reinforced. Similarly, when testing predicts that a case will be straightforward but a failed intubation follows intravenous induction of anaesthesia and paralysis, this again reinforces the idea that testing is futile. The disadvantages of testing are thus easy for the anaesthetist to see.

4.6 Why bedside airway assessment is useful

A positive test result is predicting increased likelihood of difficulty (it doesn't guarantee it). Every year a significant number of patients have their operations postponed following failed intubation and are exposed to the risks (minor and serious) of the anaesthetist encountering difficulty with airway management after induction of anaesthesia.

Although testing will miss cases, for each case that is identified the patient is not exposed to these risks. If the incidence of unanticipated airway problems is reduced by 50% there will be an equal reduction in the incidence of associated complications.

Detractors of airway assessment cite false alarms as a major problem. This is not the case if you have alternative management strategies, as the only consequence of a false alarm is the use of an alternative technique that you are comfortable with.

Assessing the airway preoperatively will allow you to choose the most appropriate and safest management technique, along with back-up plans, extra equipment, anaesthetic and surgical help that may be required.

4.7 Three recommended clinical tests

The following three clinical tests have been described in research papers with more than one grade or 'distance'. In clinical usage a single cut off point can be chosen as the decision making point at which patients are treated as 'expected to be difficult'.

4.7.1 The Mallampati test

With the patient seated ask them to open their mouth as wide as they can and stick their tongue out as far as they can (without saying 'Aah'). Inspect the oropharynx using a pen torch.

If the posterior pharyngeal wall is not visible predict difficulty with tracheal intubation with a Macintosh laryngoscope (Figure 4.3).

Figure 4.3 View at Mallampati test

(a)

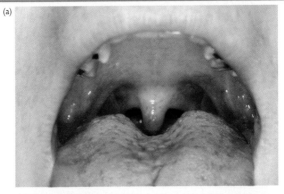

(b)

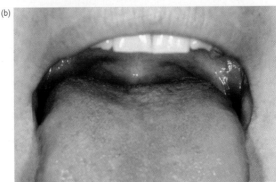

Top (a): posterior pharyngeal wall visible – more likely to be easy.
Bottom (b): posterior pharyngeal wall not visible – more likely to be difficult.

4.7.2 **Thyromental distance**

Ask the patient to tip their head back as far as they can (with their mouth closed). Measure the distance from the tip of the chin to the prominence of the thyroid cartilage.

If it is 7 cm or less, predict difficulty with tracheal intubation with a Macintosh laryngoscope (Figure 4.4).

4.7.3 **Mandibular subluxation**

Ask the patient to push their bottom teeth out in front of their top teeth.

If they are unable to do this predict difficulty with tracheal intubation with a Macintosh laryngoscope (Figure 4.5).

Single cut off points can be chosen for any airway screening test described, however we must accept that none will be correct 100% of the time.

4.8 **Combining predictive tests**

Combinations of tests have the potential to reduce false positive and false negative results and improve the overall performance of preoperative assessment. If we take as an example combining the Mallampati test and the mandibular subluxation test: The Mallampati test evaluates the size of the tongue in relation to the size of the oral cavity (the bigger the tongue the more difficult it is to displace it out of the line of sight with a laryngoscope). Mandibular subluxation evaluates how far the tongue can be lifted anteriorly out of the line of sight to the larynx. With a poor Mallampati score it may be possible to displace the tongue out of the line of sight if the jaw can be lifted a long way forward. With limited subluxation it may be possible to see past the tongue if it is small in

---

Figure 4.4 Thyromental distance

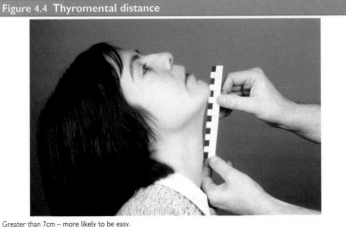

Greater than 7cm – more likely to be easy.

Figure 4.5 **Mandibular subluxation**

(a)

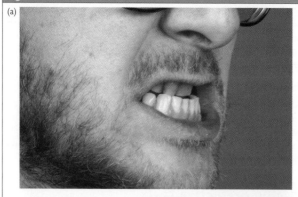

(b)

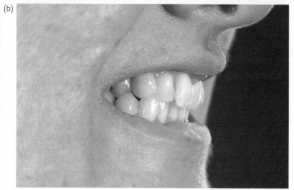

Top (a): lower incisors can be moved in front of the uppers – more likely to be easy.
Bottom (b): lower incisors cannot be moved in front of the uppers – more likely to be difficult.

relation to the size of the oral cavity. If, however, the patient has a poor Mallampati score and limited subluxation then it is highly likely that Macintosh laryngoscopy will not expose the larynx.

4.9 Using predictive tests in clinical practice

Any screening test should be followed by a decision that is informed by its result. If the result is not going to influence subsequent management there is no value in performing the test. For the purposes of airway testing this means that the anaesthetist must have an alternative airway management strategy and use it if preoperative airway assessment suggests difficult laryngoscopy.

By the same token if any of mask ventilation, LMA placement, fibreoptic intubation or surgical access to the airway are predicted difficult then they should be removed from the airway management plan or a realistic and workable action plan made for failure.

If history, examination or testing predicts difficult laryngoscopy but easy mask ventilation you need other tools available to assist with tracheal intubation. If, however, difficult ventilation is predicted, awake intubation should be chosen.

4.10 So what should I do?

Always take a history from the patient asking about problems with previous anaesthetics and review any previous anaesthetic charts for airway difficulties. The patients may carry a letter or wear a medic alert bracelet. If a previous anaesthetist had trouble with oxygenation or tracheal intubation you must devise appropriate airway management plans and choose a technique that will manage the airway safely.

There may be clues in the history that indicate difficulty with the airway including voice change, respiratory noises (stridor) and positional effects on breathing. These help to identify patients with clinical upper airway obstruction (Chapter 6).

Other general assessments should include evaluation of any concurrent medical disease process that may affect the airway. These may be local problems such as tumours, goitre or other mass distorting the airway, previous head and neck surgery or radiotherapy. For many of these, especially if symptomatic, it is useful to look for ENT reports of flexible nasendoscopy and CT and MRI scans which may help identify stenosis or deviation of the airway.

Systemic diseases known to be associated with airway management and tracheal intubation problems include rheumatoid and seronegative arthritis, ankylosing spondylitis, acromegaly, obstructive sleep apnoea, and diabetes. In many of these, the airway difficulties are anticipated by simply 'eyeballing' the patient. It is important to further distinguish these patients with anatomical problems into ones' with and without clinical upper airway obstruction. This distinction is important for safe airway management (Chapters 5 and 6).

If no previous anaesthetic history is available or the airway is not obviously grossly difficult with the 'eyeball' test then you should perform bedside airway tests. If you have your own tests that you use then continue to use them, or you may choose to modify them based on your new understanding of risk.

If you do not have a routine of your own then you may choose to use the following recipes as long as you understand their limitations.

4.11 Macintosh laryngoscopy

Perform three bedside tests (as described earlier in the chapter): Mallampati test, Thyromental distance and Mandibular protrusion. If two out of three of these tests predict difficulty then treat the patient as if Macintosh laryngoscopy is known to be difficult. Otherwise treat them as normal. Doing this will perhaps pick up half of difficult intubations (it will also miss about half of them so don't be discouraged). As with any regime there will be some false alarms. If you really don't want to miss difficult cases then you can move the cut off criteria, expecting and accepting more false alarms.

4.12 Facemask ventilation

A history of obstructive sleep apnoea, obesity, having a big beard, being edentulous and being difficult to intubate are all risk factors for difficulty with facemask ventilation.

4.13 Laryngeal masks

The only factor reliably known to make LMA use difficult is limited mouth opening. It has been suggested that with less than 20–25 mm mouth opening you should not rely on being able to use a laryngeal mask as part of your airway management strategy.

4.14 Surgical airway

This final step in the failed airway management algorithm is not always possible. In fixed flexion neck deformity or where there is local infection or marked swelling a surgical airway may not be available as a rescue technique. Therefore the suitability for cricothyroidotomy should be assessed at the pre-operative evaluation and not assumed available.

4.15 Fibreoptic intubation

An awake technique is more likely to be utilized if there are several factors pointing to difficulty. However, no technique is 100% effective, even in expert hands. The predictors for difficulty in fibreoptic intubation are different from direct laryngoscopy and include blood or secretions in the airway and significant reduction in the size of the laryngeal inlet (Chapter 6). Other factors such as patient compliance, choice of tracheal tube and experience of the operator also play a part (Chapter 7).

Using this knowledge to predict airway difficulty at the bedside will help avoid most unplanned can't intubate and can't ventilate scenarios, which can be very costly for the patient and the anaesthetist alike. Remember false negatives and false positives are a part of any test. False positives will only mean you use a safe alternative technique that allows you to gain another skill for your airway armamentarium under controlled circumstances. If you have assessed the airway for the suitability for different management strategies you should be able to safely work your way down the difficult airway algorithm when a false positive or false negative is encountered.

Further reading

Darshane S, Groom P, Charters P. Responsive contingency planning: a novel system for anticipated difficulty in airway management in dental abscess. *British Journal of Anaesthesia* 2007; **99**: 898–905.

Greenland KB. A proposed model for direct laryngoscopy and tracheal intubation, *Anaesthesia* 2008; **63**: 156–61.

Kheterpal S, Han R, Tremper KK, Shanks A, Tait AR, O'Reilly M, Ludwig TA. Incidence and predictors of difficult and impossible mask ventilation. *Anesthesiology* 2006; **105**: 885–91.

Loong TW. Understanding sensitivity and specificity with the right side of the brain, *British Medical Journal* 2003; **327**: 716–19.

Law M. Screening without evidence of efficacy, *British Medical Journal* 2004; **328**: 301–2.

Cortellazzi, P, Minati, L, Falcone, C, Lamperti, M and Caldiroli, D. Predictive value of the El-Ganzouri multivariate risk index for difficult tracheal intubation: a comparison of Glidescope ® videolaryngoscopy and conventional Macintosh laryngoscopy. *British Journal of Anaesthesia* 2007; **99**: 906–11.

Chapter 5

Management of the anticipated difficult airway: without clinical upper airway obstruction

Mike Goodwin

Key points

- Recognition and planning is the key to success
- There should be at least one back up plan thought out in *advance*
- To execute each plan, use of procedures with which you are familiar, rather than experimentation is more likely to result in success
- The overriding principle is to avoid progression to a 'can't intubate, can't ventilate' situation
- General anaesthesia can easily induce airway obstruction and its life threatening consequences in these patients
- For this reason securing the airway using an 'awake' technique such as awake fibreoptic intubation remains as the gold standard of management in these patients.

5.1 Introduction

The anticipated difficult airway scenario *without clinical upper airway obstruction* conforms well to the 5 'P' scheme discussed in Chapter 2. The key to the management of the anticipated difficult airway is in its recognition (the first 'P' – preoperative assessment), in order that a safe management strategy may be planned (the second 'P' – planning') for each individual patient. For each step (the third 'P' – procedure) there needs to be a back-up plan should problems be encountered, in order to minimize the possibility of progression to a 'can't intubate, can't ventilate' (CICV) scenario. It must be remembered that extubation of the patient with an anticipated difficult airway may also be difficult and this should be planned (the fourth 'P' – post procedure). Finally, immaculate records of the events would help in the future care of the patient and if appropriate measures should be taken to arrange for an airway alert (the fifth 'P' – publicity).

It must be borne in mind that in some cases, despite a meticulous assessment of the patient's airway, difficulty arises unexpectedly and anaesthetists must be prepared to manage this scenario (Chapter 8).

This chapter deals only with situations where difficulty is known of, or is anticipated due to anatomical and/or pathological factors and there is *no evidence of clinical upper airway obstruction.* Patients presenting with clinical airway obstruction are dealt with in Chapter 6.

Examples of patients with anticipated difficult airway (no airway obstruction) are shown as a slide show – www.orag.co.uk/book.

5.2 Recognition (pre operative assessment)

Recognition of possible difficulties with face mask ventilation, direct laryngoscopy and intubation is sometimes simple because the airway is obviously grossly abnormal (the eyeball test) due to disease, surgery or radiotherapy. It is worth remembering that difficulties may be associated with certain congenital syndromes (Chapter 11) and certain acquired conditions such as obesity, pregnancy, trauma, infection, tumour and arthropathies (e.g. ankylosing spondylitis, rheumatoid arthritis), previous surgery and radiotherapy to head and neck area.

Recognition in less obvious cases depends upon previous good record keeping, history taking, clinical examination, and radiological investigations. There is no single clinical test with a sufficiently high sensitivity and specificity to reliably detect all difficult airways whilst excluding all straightforward ones, so a number of factors are employed in shaping one's clinical judgment (see Chapter 4). It is useful to be able to answer the following questions at the end of the pre operative assessment:

- Is face mask ventilation going to be difficult?
- Is supraglottic airway insertion/ventilation going to be difficult?
- Is tracheal intubation going to be difficult? This not only includes direct laryngoscopy but also other alternative techniques if they are part of the airway management plan
- Is the patient suitable for an 'awake' intubation?
- Is surgical access to the airway going to be difficult?

5.3 Planning

Once it has been established that management of the airway is going to be 'difficult' then planning should include the following considerations:

1. Can surgery be safely performed under local/regional anaesthesia?
2. If the patient needs a general anaesthetic then the gold standard is to secure the airway while the patient is awake by 'awake' tracheal intubation.
3. Alternative intubation plans should be considered in cases where awake intubation is desirable but is not feasible or is contraindicated (see below).
4. It may be possible to conduct surgery with a supra glottic device with the patient breathing spontaneously or even paralysed.
5. A small minority of patient may require a surgical airway as Plan A.

5.3.1 Surgery can be safely performed under local/regional anaesthesia

The following conditions must be fulfilled when surgery is contemplated under local/regional anaesthesia in a patient with a known difficult airway:

1. Surgery should be feasible under local/regional block, e.g. limb surgery, obstetric and gynaecological surgery.
2. The airway must be accessible at all times.
3. A back up airway management plan should always be worked out in advance and communicated to the patient, anaesthetic assistant, and surgeon.
4. The anaesthetist must be experienced in performing both the regional anaesthesia technique and also in rescuing the airway should problems occur.

5.3.2 If the patient needs a general anaesthetic then the priority should be to secure the airway by tracheal intubation while the patient is awake

Tracheal intubation is the most definitive way to secure airway patency, ensure adequate ventilation and prevent aspiration of gastric contents. In the patient with a known/anticipated difficult airway it is considered 'gold standard' to secure the airway by awake intubation. Almost all patients even those in the advanced stages of the conditions listed above have the ability to breathe when awake It is only when anaesthesia is induced that airway obstruction becomes a problem and that manoeuvres involving the laryngoscope prove to be of restricted use. The logical conclusion is that all risks to these patients arise from induction of anaesthesia. Therefore, it seems further logical to secure the airway of patients identified to be potentially difficult airways when these patients are awake and before induction of general anaesthesia.

Advantages of awake tracheal intubation

- Natural airway is preserved, spontaneous breathing allows adequate ventilation.
- Airway is protected from aspiration of gastric contents.
- Neurological monitoring after intubation if required.

- Cardiovascular stability.
- Safe back up plan.
- Good for your coronaries!

Several techniques can be used to secure the airway by awake intubation and these are discussed below (see Procedures).

5.3.3 Alternative intubation plans should be considered in cases where awake intubation is desirable but is not feasible or is contraindicated

Examples of this scenario can occur in the following:

- paediatric patients;
- patients with learning disabilities;
- uncooperative patients (e.g. head injury, intoxication);
- massive haemorrhage in upper airway;
- local anaesthetic hypersensitivity;
- where consent is withheld.

When general anaesthesia is contemplated in a patient with an anticipated difficult airway, further considerations should include

  i. Method of induction of anaesthesia: Inhalation versus Intravenous.
  ii. Method of intubation: in the spontaneously breathing patient or in the paralysed patient.

The techniques that can be used to facilitate intubation in this group of patients are summarized below (see procedures).

5.3.4 It may be possible to conduct surgery with a supra glottic device with the patient breathing spontaneously or even paralysed

Many surgical procedures can be safely performed with a supra glottic device, usually a laryngeal mask airway. It is possible to avoid tracheal intubation in these cases. If this decision is undertaken then it is absolutely vital to ascertain that face mask ventilation and insertion of supra glottic device are not predicted to be difficult. Decisions have also to be made of whether the patient is allowed to breathe spontaneously or whether ventilation is controlled with the supra glottic device. A strategy to secure the airway with a tracheal tube should always be in place should problems occur. The formulation of this back up (Plan B) in this situation cannot be over emphasised. The anaesthetist concerned should be experienced in performing this 'back up' technique and the necessary equipment should be readily available.

5.3.5 A small minority of patients may require a surgical airway.

5.4 **Procedures (the third 'P')**

This section deals with the techniques that may be used to execute the above airway management plans.

5.4.1 **Awake intubation**

Although commonly referred to as 'awake' these techniques are often facilitated by judicious conscious sedation in most cases.

5.4.2 **Techniques of 'awake' intubation**

- Awake flexible fibreoptic intubation (oral or nasal).
- Awake intubation using supra glottic device (e.g. laryngeal mask, intubating laryngeal mask).
- Awake retrograde intubation (with or without fibreoptic guidance).
- Awake direct laryngoscopy.
- Awake blind nasal intubation.

5.4.2.1 *Awake flexible fibreoptic intubation (oral or nasal)*

The use of the flexible fibreoptic scope for awake intubation has revolutionized the management of the patient with an anticipated difficult airway. Proper preparation is essential for success. The techniques are detailed in Chapter 7.

5.4.2.2 *Awake intubation using supra glottic device (e.g. laryngeal mask, intubating laryngeal mask)*

The use of both the standard and intubating laryngeal mask has been described to facilitate intubation in awake patients. The devices are surprisingly very well tolerated and provide an excellent conduit to guide the tube to the laryngeal inlet. These devices may be particularly useful in the presence of blood and/or secretions in the oral cavity where a 'direct' fibreoptic technique may be difficult. The success rate of blind intubation through supraglottic devices is low and and there is a real risk of trauma to the upper airway. Therefore a technique using fibreoptic guidance is recommended.

5.4.2.3 *Awake retrograde intubation (with or without fibreoptic guidance)*

Indications for this technique include patients with gross distortion of the upper airway anatomy. Direct nasal or oral fibreoptic are predicted to be difficult. The technique involves inserting a wire or epidural catheter guided upwards through a cricothyroid puncture. This is then grasped in the mouth or nose. The options then are to insert a tube directly over the wire (may be difficult) or insert a Cook exchange catheter over the wire first and railroad the tube over the exchange catheter. Alternatively the insertion cord of a flexible fibreoptic scope can be inserted over the wire, advanced until it reaches the trachea and then a tube can be railroaded over the fibrescope.

5.4.2.4 *Awake direct laryngoscopy*

This is now only used in the extremes when other techniques are not feasible. A previously very useful technique was to perform an 'awake look' direct laryngoscopy. This involved inserting a Macintosh laryngoscope blade in the oral cavity after establishing local anaesthesia of the upper airway. If any part of the epiglottis was visible then the patient would be induced and intubation accomplished under general anaesthesia.

5.4.2.5 *Awake blind nasal intubation*

This useful technique was commonly used but has now been superseded by flexible fibreoptic techniques.

5.4.3 Alternative intubation techniques where awake intubation is desirable but is not feasible or is contraindicated:

- Decide the merits of induction of anaesthesia with inhalation versus intravenous agents.
- Decide the merits of intubation in the paralysed versus spontaneously breathing patient.

The following is a suggested list of techniques. The choice would depend on the circumstances with the patient, the availability of equipment, and the experience of the anaesthetist. Some of these techniques are detailed in Chapters 8 and 11 and the use of some of the newer devices and techniques is described in Chapter 13.

- Direct laryngoscopy – optimization with Macintosh laryngoscope and bougie.
- Use of alternative blades, e.g. McCoy, Straight.
- Indirect laryngoscope, e.g. Airtraq, Glidescope, Mcgrath.
- Rigid fibreoptic scope, e.g. Bullard, Wu scope.
- Optical stylets, e.g. Levitan, Shikani.
- Blind intubation through intubating laryngeal mask.
- Flexible fibreoptic guided intubation through intubating laryngeal mask.
- Flexible fibreoptic guided intubation through other supra glottic airway, e.g. laryngeal mask (with or without Aintree catheter).
- Direct flexible fibreoptic intubation – nasal or oral route.
- Retrograde intubation with or without fibreoptic guidance.
- Blind nasal intubation.

5.5 Prophylactic cricothyroid cannula

More recently some anaesthetists are inserting a 'prophylactic' cannula through the cricothyroid membrane before performing the planned techniques, e.g. awake fibreoptic intubation. This allows to secure oxygenation via a jet ventilation device should problems occur with the planned primary technique.

Further Reading

Please refer to **www.orag.co.uk/book** for slide show of examples of patients with anticipated difficult airway. Slides show recognition, planning and some procedures.

An Updated Report by the ASA Task Force on Management of the Difficult Airway. Practice guidelines for the management of the difficult airway. *Anesthesiology* 2003; **98**: 1269–77.

Benumof JL. Management of the difficult airway: with special emphasis on awake tracheal intubation. *Anesthesiology* 1991; **75**: 1087–1110.

Benumof JL. ASA Difficult Airway Algorithm: New Thought and Considerations. In: *Handbook of Difficult Airway Management.* Hagberg CA. ed. Churchill Livingstone Philadelphia 2000; 31–48.

Charters P and O'Sullivan E. The 'dedicated airway': a review of the concept and an update of current practice. *Anaesthesia* 1999; **54**: 778–86.

Gerig HJ, Schnider T, Heidegger T. Prophylactic percutaneous transtracheal catheterisation in the management of patients with anticipated difficult airways: a case series. *Anaesthesia.* 2005; **60**: 801–5.

Ovassapian A. Fibreoptic Tracheal Intubation in Adults. In: Ovassapian A. ed. *Fibreoptic Endoscopy and the Difficult Airway.* Philadelphia, Lippincot-Raven 1996 72–103.

Popat M. State of the art. The airway. *Anaesthesia* 2003; **58**: 1166–72.

Chapter 6

Management of the anticipated difficult airway: the patient with critical upper airway obstruction

Stuart W. Benham

Key points

- Recognize that critical upper airway obstruction is present
- Clinical evaluation is most important in determining the site, severity and progress of the obstruction
- A scheme based on the need for intervention scenarios – immediate, urgent or non-urgent is used to understand the airway management principles
- Immediate basic life support and definitive control of the airway are paramount for management of the immediate scenario
- The site, severity and extent of the obstruction determine the airway management techniques that can be used for the urgent and non-urgent scenario
- The involvement of senior personnel, surgical back up and expert anaesthetic assistance is vital to safe patient management.

6.1 Introduction

The term 'upper airway obstruction' is used in this chapter to describe a variety of clinical situations in which airway compromise, if untreated, threatens life. Conditions associated with distortion of upper airway anatomy resulting in anticipated airway difficulties but not causing airway obstruction are dealt with in Chapter 5. The purpose of this chapter is to summarize the causes of acute upper airway obstruction (Box 6.1), outline the general principles of airway evaluation and present guidelines for safe management.

Box 6.1 Common causes of upper airway obstruction

A. Acute obstruction in a previously 'normal airway':

- Unconsciousness from any cause
- Laryngeal spasm during anaesthesia
- Angioneurotic oedema
- Trauma to the face and upper airway
- Foreign body in the upper airway
- Infection in and around the upper airway
- *(Ludwig's angina, tonsillar abscess, epiglottitis)*
- Burn and thermal injury
- Post surgical neck haematoma

The above scenarios may occur in a matter of minutes or hours in a previously normal airway. The underlying oedema, pus or blood in the upper airway tissues is responsible and therefore this obstruction is 'fluidic' in nature and stridor may be an early presenting feature.

B. Chronic airway compromise presenting as acute upper airway obstruction:

- Benign lesions and malignant tumours in the upper airway
  Supraglottic: floor of mouth, tongue, pharynx,
  Glottic and periglottic: Epiglottic, pyriform fossa, vocal cords
  Subglottic: upper tracheal, thyroid goitre
  Mid tracheal/bronchial: mediastinal masses
- Previous surgery for any of the above
- Previous radiotherapy in the head and neck area for any of the above

Chronic upper airway compromise usually occurs over a matter of weeks or months. It is due to tumour mass or fibrosis and is therefore 'solid' in nature. Stridor is usually a late presenting feature and is due to extensive disease, bleeding or infection in the tumour. The underlying anatomical abnormalities may make mask ventilation, laryngeal mask insertion, and/or direct laryngoscopy difficult.

In managing upper airway obstruction from any cause, the fact that the airway is already compromised means that a safe approach is to prioritize maintaining ventilation although compromised, while executing plan(s) to secure a definitive airway.

6.2 **Recognizing obstruction**

If airway assessment is a core skill for all anaesthetists, recognizing a compromised airway that could lead to life threatening upper airway obstruction must be considered one of the most important aspects of this skill.

I recall as a junior anaesthetist being asked to attend a patient in the Emergency Department who had been there for hours with suspected epiglottitis and his airway becoming increasingly compromised. The moment I arrived, his respiratory distress was well advanced, and he was peri-arrest. His imminent collapse prevented any airway workup, and his respiratory arrest required an emergency surgical airway. Here lack of recognition of a compromised airway led to a potentially unnecessary surgical intervention, when a more deliberate and planned work-up could have secured the airway without the need to resort to a scalpel.

6.2.1 History and clinical examination

Although anaesthetists will encounter some very rapidly advancing emergencies, most cases of upper airway obstruction allow time for planning the safest method of securing the airway, with the appropriate people in attendance. History and clinical examination are most important and the key questions are:

1. Is upper airway obstruction present? If yes, what is its site, extent, and severity?
2. How rapidly is it progressing?

The symptoms and signs of upper airway obstruction are due to

- increased work of breathing;
- ineffective ventilation;
- secondary effects of hypoxia/hypercapnia.

Increased work of breathing causes an increase in respiratory rate (tachypnoea); see saw breathing with intercostal and substernal muscle recession and use of accessory muscles of respiration.

Stridor, when it is present, is due to narrowing of the airway lumen causing the normal laminar flow through the upper airway to be replaced by turbulent flow (noisy breathing) due to increased negative pressure in the upper airway. It has been suggested that the airway diameter is reduced by 50% when stridor is present. The difficulty is in determining how much more than this the airway is obstructed. With moderate obstruction, stridor is present on exertion; stridor at rest indicates critical airway narrowing. The respiratory phase during which stridor occurs may indicate the site of obstruction; inspiratory stridor indicating lesions at or above the vocal cords; expiratory stridor indicating lesions below the vocal cords.

With progressive obstruction, signs of ineffective ventilation and poor gas exchange (hypoxia and hypercapnia) are present. These include cyanosis and altered level of consciousness presenting as agitation, anxiety, confusion or restlessness. Secondary effects of hypoxia and hypercapnia such as tachycardia, hypertension, and sweating may also be present.

In late stages, not only does the patient complain of noisy breathing (stridor), but also of difficulty in breathing, often preferring to sit up and waking up at night to get fresh air. Pharyngeal involvement is indicated by difficulty in swallowing and clearing secretions, dyphonia and hoarseness suggest that the larynx is involved.

Complete airway obstruction may present with unconsciousness, a silent chest, slow respiratory rate and bradycardia.

6.2.2 Airway assessment and investigations

Forewarned is forearmed when dealing with airway obstruction. *As a minimum, routine assessment to highlight potential difficulty with mask ventilation and/or direct laryngoscopy must be carried out.* This has an important bearing on the management techniques (see below)

In some cases of acute airway obstruction, investigations are not desirable for fear of exacerbating the condition (e.g. epiglottitis, post operative haematoma, angioneurotic oedema) or when measures to oxygenate the patient and establishing adequate ventilation are a priority. In all other cases, investigations are performed to complement the history and physical examination.

The following three investigations, depending on the severity and cause of the obstruction, are most important:

- Indirect laryngoscopy and/or flexible fibreoptic nasendoscopy are performed to determine if the vocal cords are seen and if a tracheal tube will pass the narrow glottis or not.
- MRI/CT of the upper airway from the mouth to the trachea is useful to determine the extent and cause of the obstruction. It may also reveal tumour dissemination and other areas of obstruction missed on clinical examination.
- Blood gases to determine hypoxia/hypercapnia.

The following may be performed if time or condition of the patient permits:

- Chest X-ray to determine airway diameter, tracheal deviation, extrinsic compression.
- ECG may reveal right ventricular hypertrophy and strain in chronic cases.
- Soft tissue radiographs of the head and neck.
- Pulmonary function tests with flow volume loops may help in determining the site of obstruction.

6.3 **Management of upper airway obstruction**

This can be discussed under three scenarios – immediate, urgent, and non-urgent. This distinction is for clarity only and in practice a patient can very rapidly move from an urgent scenario to an immediate one.

1. When immediate action is required – within minutes.
2. When urgent action is required – within hours.
3. When non urgent action is required (stable obstruction) – within days.

6.3.1 **When immediate action is required**

Most cases of acute upper airway obstruction are triggered by trauma, bleeding or oedema in a previously normal airway (Box 6.1). Examples in this category include angioneurotic oedema, laryngeal spasm, foreign body or severe trauma to the upper airway. In life threatening situations, basic life support to provide oxygen and ensure a patent airway should be instituted while preparations are made for definitive control of the airway. Pulse, blood pressure, and oxygen saturation need to be monitored. A calm and reassuring approach from health professionals minimizes the anxiety of the situation (despite what you may feel inside). Recognize the gravity of the situation, and that imminent loss of upper airway is likely. All senior staff – surgeon, senior anaesthetist, and senior ODP must be summoned without delay. Specific measures to treat the underlying condition e.g. nebulized adrenaline and steroids for angioneurotic oedema should be instituted as soon as possible.

6.3.1.1 *Airway management*

A rapid upper airway assessment to identify any suggestion that direct laryngoscopy would be difficult is essential to implement the plan for definitive airway management.

If this suggests that no additional difficulties would be expected then following 100% pre-oxygenation an intravenous induction with rapid muscle relaxation is undertaken, with the full knowledge and support of a competent surgeon standing by with all available kit at the ready to perform a surgical airway. Direct laryngoscopy in the optimized fashion is performed and a suitably sized tracheal tube is placed under direct vision. For example (facial injuries due road traffic accident) log on www.orag.co.uk/book.

If airway assessment suggests direct laryngoscopy could be difficult, then a more cautious inhalational induction with sevoflurane and 100% oxygen is delivered, until laryngoscopy can be performed before muscle relaxation. The same attention to having the surgical back-up applies.

If airway assessment suggests that mask ventilation and/or supra glottic device insertion could be difficult, then the safest course of action may be to secure the airway surgically under local infiltration. For example (facial injuries due to gun shot) log on www.orag.co.uk/book.

6.3.1.2 *Rationale for above approach*

If direct laryngoscopy is anticipated to be straight forward, then securing the airway with a tracheal tube before further ground is lost and oxygenation becomes impossible is the safest option. The intravenous induction route achieves this quickly, and direct laryngoscopy allows the best chance of securing the airway rapidly.

If there is doubt about ease of laryngoscopy, the additional time to institute anaesthesia via inhalation route is worth it, as it allows oxygenation while deepening the anaesthetic, and allows assessment of laryngoscopy before muscle relaxation.

This decision is not easy, and following either route may still fail, and lead to utilizing the rescue surgical technique.

6.3.2 **When urgent intervention is required**

Examples of this scenario include patients with post surgical neck haematoma, dental abscesses and Ludwig's angina, thermal injury and trauma to the upper airway. Occasionally a patient with chronic obstruction due to tumour may present acutely when the growth is extensive or if there is bleeding or infection in the tumour.

If expeditious measures to secure the airway are not taken, then these conditions can deteriorate into a life threatening situation (immediate scenario). The key to success is to individualize patient management based on history and clinical examination, In certain situations a clinical history and examination suffice to determine the cause of the obstruction and investigations may not be appropriate, for example in a sick patient with epiglottitis, where any disturbance is likely to make airway obstruction worse. In other cases more time is available to perform investigations (e.g. MRI scans in dental abscesses) to establish the diagnosis; plan the airway management and surgical treatment. Think through both the primary airway plan, and any back up plans, and ensure all the equipment and personnel required to carry out these plans are available before embarking on the airway management strategy. In this situation choosing the correct location for the attempt to secure the airway may be the most important decision (Emergency Room, anaesthetic room, or theatre itself).

The safe management of these patients depends on determining the site and extent (supraglottic, glottic, infraglottic, or lower tracheal) of airway obstruction because the principles of airway management are different in each of these cases.

6.3.2.1 *Supraglottic pathology*

Airway compromise is usually at the level of the oropharynx or nasopharynx and is due to mechanical obstruction caused by tumour and/or due to factors such as previous surgery, radiotherapy and bony deformities. The larynx may be deviated to one side but there is usually no direct involvement unless there is bleeding or oedema. Induction of general anaesthesia may worsen the obstruction and multiple attempts at laryngoscopy may make a manageable airway, unmanageable. For this reason, the safest approach is to secure the airway while the patient is awake usually with a flexible fibreoptic scope.

Awake fibreoptic intubation in this scenario may not be straight forward and the for it to be successful the following considerations are essential:

- Should be performed by an experienced anaesthetist with good endoscopy skills.
- Preferable to have the patient sitting upright.
- Supplemental oxygenation at all times.
- Minimal or no sedation.
- Meticulous topical anaesthesia to avoid airway irritation and spasm.
- Surgical back up ready to perform a surgical airway in the 'awake' patient.

The following examples of patients with acute upper airway obstruction requiring urgent action are shown as slides show and video clips on www.orag.co.uk/book.

Ludwig's angina, end stage supra glottic tumour with metastasis, acute post operative haematoma following surgery in the mouth.

6.3.2.2 *Periglottic and glottic obstruction*

The airway management plan depends on the findings of a preoperative nasendoscopy performed by an experienced ENT surgeon (or anaesthetist). Nasendoscopy is performed to determine the extent of the lesion and diameter of the laryngeal inlet in order to decide whether a tracheal tube can be passed through the narrowed airway. This procedure is well tolerated by most patients without any topical anaesthesia of the airway.

If nasendoscopy reveals that a small tracheal tube can be negotiated through the narrowed glottis, then the choice is between an awake fibreoptic technique and intubation after inhalation general anaesthesia using direct laryngoscopy.

An inhalation induction in these patients can be difficult and may result in complete airway obstruction. This can occur as a result of coughing in the light stages of anaesthesia or when deep anaesthesia causes relaxation of the pharyngeal muscles. The latter may be relieved with a nasopharyngeal airway inserted in a nostril previously prepared with cocaine. When anaesthesia is deep enough, gentle laryngoscopy is performed and if after one or two attempts, intubation is not possible than the surgeon, who is already gowned and ready, is asked to perform a tracheostomy with the patient breathing spontaneously (plan B).

The argument in favour of this technique is that ideal conditions for topical anaesthesia and sedation for awake fibreoptic intubation are difficult to achieve in these patients and the procedure is technically challenging. Total airway obstruction can result from topical anaesthesia itself or from the physical presence of the fibrescope in the narrowed airway (cork in the bottle phenomenon). Other factors such as performing the technique in the supine position, sedation and multiple attempts at fibreoptic endoscopy may also be responsible. This approach assumes that direct laryngoscopy is not predicted to be difficult.

My advice to anybody contemplating awake fibreoptic intubation in this scenario is to avoid sedation, perform the technique with the patient in the sitting position and avoid multiple attempts. This requires an experienced endoscopist who has the ability and confidence to deal with abnormal airway anatomy on a regular basis. The flexibility and versatility of flexible fibreoptic endoscopy allows dynamic assessment of the airway anatomy in the glottic and sub glottic region in an atraumatic fashion. This approach allows the patient to be awake and self ventilating at all times. If fibreoptic endoscopy and/or intubation fail, then a tracheostomy is performed under local anaesthesia by the surgeon who is ready and gowned (plan B).

If the initial nasendoscopy reveals a very advanced lesion suggesting that enough space is not available to negotiate a small tube, then a safe plan is for the surgeon to perform a definitive surgical airway under local anaesthesia.

6.3.2.3 *Sub glottic/Mid tracheal compression*

Airway obstruction at this level can result from pathology within the trachea (tumours, tracheal stenosis, or tracheomalacia) or external compression (thyroid). It is of vital importance in these cases to determine the site and extent (especially of the lower end) of airway narrowing by chest X-ray and gantry enhanced CT/MRI imaging. If other predictors of difficult laryngoscopy are not present, then most of these patients can be intubated with conventional direct laryngoscopy. The problem with this approach is that it is uncertain if the tip of the tracheal tube will go past the obstruction and lie beyond the obstruction. For this reason a flexible fibreoptic endoscopy performed in the awake patient will allow dynamic airway assessment and tube selection and will ensure that the distal end of the tube is beyond the obstruction. Another option is to place a size 7 mm tracheal tube above the obstruction, and using it as a conduit for passing a Jet Ventilation catheter beyond the obstruction. This is a valid plan for those practitioners who use this form of ventilation routinely, but not for the novice. The requirement for an adequate route for exhalation is mandatory when employing jet ventilation. Ignoring this can lead to severe barotrauma, worsening hypoxia and respiratory arrest. Where the obstruction is likely to hamper placement of even a small size tube, the recommendation is for prophylactic placement of femoral arterio-venous vascular access to allow patient to be placed on extra corporeal oxygenation circuit. The patient is anaesthetized in the cardiac theatres with the pump technicians primed and ready to connect to the circuit, should partial obstruction deteriorate to inadequate oxygenation. This plan is chosen because a surgical airway in the form of tracheostomy may be difficult to impossible in patients with a large mass in the neck..

6.3.2.4 *Lower tracheal and bronchial obstruction*

The common causes are mediastinal masses and vascular lesions. If the obstruction is lower down in the trachea then general anaesthesia is extremely dangerous as it will lead to loss of muscle tone and tracheal collapse. For this reason, the ideal management of such patients is in a cardiothoracic centre with facilities for cardiopulmonary by-pass and expertise in rigid bronchoscopy.

6.3.3 **When non urgent action is required (stable obstruction) – within days**

The upper airway obstruction is due to pathology above the glottis, at or near the glottis or below the glottis. In this scenario the upper airway is compromised but not to an extent where surgical intervention is urgently needed. The symptoms usually point to this. For example, a patient with a big tumour in the supra glottic region or a patient with a malignant goitre having stridor when lying down but not when sitting up. There are also patients with 'fixed' obstruction for example due to tracheal narrowing due to fibrosis, who repeatedly have laser surgery.

The management principles of dealing with obstruction at different anatomical levels in these patients are similar to that discussed under the urgent scenario (see above). The difference is that more time is available for planning and often these patients are operated on during an elective surgical list.

The following examples of patients with stable obtrution requiring non urgent intervention are shown in **www.orag.co.uk/book**:

- Supraglottic obstrtion due to tumour, surgery, radiothearapy. Slide and videoclip.
- Infraglottic obstruction due to thyroid goiter.

6.3.4 **Prophylactic placement of cricothyroidotomy cannula**

This extremely useful and relatively simple technique provides a route for rescue oxygenation in the event of worsening hypoxaemia during performance of a definitive airway management technique. The procedure involves inserting a dedicated narrow bore cannula (e.g. Ravussin) through the cricothyroid membrane under local anaesthesia before performing the definitive technique. The rationale being that the cannula can be used to provide jet ventilation and thereby oxygenate the patient should problems occur. This procedure requires experience and may be difficult to perform in the patient with a rapidly deteriorating upper airway. It should not delay the definitive airway management procedures outlined above. A dedicated high pressure ventilator (e.g. Manujet) should be available.

The guidance given in this chapter is to help the anaesthetist understand the principles of airway management in the patient with upper airway obstruction. Many specialist units deal with a particular subset of these patients. Their experience and set up allows them to use techniques which may not be considered 'conventional' by others.

Further reading

Calder I and Koh KF. Cervical haematoma and airway obstruction. *Br J Anaesth* 1996; **76**: 888.

Cheney FW, Posner KL, Caplan RA. Adverse respiratory events infrequently leading to malpractice suits. A closed claims analysis. *Anesthesiology* 1991; **75**: 932–9.

Gray AJG, Hoile RW, Ingram GS, Sherry KM. The obstructed airway in head and neck surgery. *The report of the National Confidential Enquiry into Perioperative Deaths* 1996/1997: 27–32.

Ho AMH, Chung DC, To EWH, et al. Total airway obstruction during local anesthesia in a non-sedated patient with a compromised airway. *Can J Anaesth* 2004; **51**: 838–41.

Mason RA, Fielder CP. The obstructed airway in head and neck surgery. *Anaesthesia* 1999; **54**: 625–8.

McGuire G and El-Beheory H. Complete airway obstruction during awake fibreoptic intubation in patients with unstable cervical spine fractures. *Can J Aneth* 1999; **46**: 176–8.

Moore EW, Davies MW. Inhalational versus intravenous induction. A survey of emergency anaesthetic practice in the United Kingdom. *European Journal of Anesthesiology* 2000; **17**: 33–7.

Popat M, Dudnikov S. Management of the obstructed upper airway. In *Current Anaesthesia and Critical Care. Focus on Difficult Airway*, ed Pollard BJ. Harcourt Publishers Ltd, London 2001; **12**: 225–30.

Shaw IC, Welchew EA, Harrison BJ, Michael S. Complete airway obstruction during awake fibreoptic intubation. *Anaesthesia* 1997; **52**: 582–5.

Chapter 7

Awake fibreoptic intubation

Mansukh Popat and Mridula Rai

> **Key points**
> - Awake fibreoptic intubation is the gold standard for intubation in a patient with an anticipated difficult airway
> - Proper planning and execution with attention to detail are keys to patient compliance and a high success rate
> - Good endoscopy technique, meticulous topical anaesthesia of the upper airway, conscious sedation, and the correct choice of tube and railroading techniques are vital to the success of this technique.

7.1 Introduction

The role of awake intubation in the management of the anticipated difficult airway scenario has been described in Chapters 5 and 6. The flexible fibreoptic scope has unique advantages in an awake intubation (Box 7.1) and is an important tool in the anaesthetists' armamentarium. This chapter deals with some 'practical' aspects of awake fibre optic intubation and useful tips to ensure success.

Awake fibreoptic intubation may not be an appropriate technique in the following situations:

- inexperience of the operator in performing the technique;
- most children;

> **Box 7.1 Advantages of the flexible fibreoptic scope for awake intubation**
> - Flexibility and continuous visualization allows one to negotiate even the most difficult anatomy.
> - Can be used for oral and nasal intubation.
> - Can be used with other devices, e.g. LMA/ILMA to aid intubation.
> - Ability to apply local anaesthetic through working channel is unique.
> - Immediate definitive tube position check.
> - Applicable to all age groups.
> - Excellent patient acceptability.
> - Very high success rate.

- uncooperative adults, e.g. learning disability, altered consciousness level;
- patient's refusal;
- local anaesthetic sensitivity;
- massive haemorrhage in the mouth.

Proper planning and execution with attention to detail are keys to patient compliance and a high success rate. These are discussed under the following headings. It is assumed that the operator has been taught fibreoptic dexterity skills on off patient models and gained experience in using the fibrescope in anaesthetized patients.

1. Airway evaluation
2. Include back up plan
3. Explanation and consent
4. Premedication
5. Monitoring (also sedation)
6. Oxygenation
7. Conscious sedation
8. Upper airway local anaesthesia
9. Good endoscopy technique
10. Choice of tube and technique of railroading

7.2 Airway evaluation

Two questions need to be answered:

1. Does the patient need an awake intubation?

The preoperative assessment (Chapters 2, 4) would determine whether the patient is suitable for an awake intubation.

2. Is the awake fibreoptic intubation going to be easy or difficult?

In our experience of both performing and teaching over 800 awake fibreoptic intubations, we have made the following observations.

For pictures and video of patients and techniques log on to www.orag.co.uk/book.

7.2.1 **Patients with only bony anatomical problems**

Examples which include TMJ ankylosis and ankylosing spondylitis would be predicted to be difficult to intubate with conventional direct laryngoscopy but are generally easy to intubate awake using the flexible fibreoptic scope.

7.2.2 **Patients with some degree of soft tissue airway pathology, with or without bony abnormality but with no clinical signs and symptoms of upper airway obstruction**

These patients would generally be easy but may occasionally be difficult due to the presence of the 'bulk' of the tumour or as a result of previous surgery.

Blood and secretions may be present and can make topical anaesthesia difficult. A novice operator may find these situations quite challenging.

7.2.3 **Patients with soft tissue pathology and presenting with clinical signs of upper airway obstruction (stridor)**

These are the most difficult. There is a real risk of complete airway obstruction (cork in the bottle situation) due to narrowed airway. Each patient has to be assessed individually and in some cases an awake fibreoptic intubation may be contraindicated. Sedation is ideally avoided and the anaesthetist performing the procedure must be an accomplished 'endoscopist'.

7.3 **Include back up plan**

Never assume that an AFI would always be successful and it is vital to have a back up plan. This may involve utilizing the expertise of a senior colleague or a surgeon.

7.4 **Explanation and consent**

A thorough, unhurried explanation of the technique should then follow. We find it is useful to explain to the patient what is intubation, why is it indicated, and how would it usually be performed in a patient with a normal airway. Then explain the difficulties that would result if intubation were to be performed after induction of anaesthesia and the safety of an awake fibreoptic technique in their case. Reassure the patient that they do not have to be wide awake during the procedure but will be sedated and comfortable and that a significant proportion of patients have no recall of the event afterwards.

The local anaesthetic technique is explained carefully and the patient is warned that this will reduce the discomfort of the procedure but not provide complete numbness. It is also important to mention that railroading the tube may sometimes be uncomfortable. It is easy to liken the procedure to an upper gastrointestinal endoscopy (with which many patients are familiar) emphasizing that the intubating fibrescope is a much thinner tube. The patient is reassured that they will have a general anaesthetic once the tracheal tube is in place. This conversation is not only an explanation of the procedure but also more importantly helps to establish a rapport with the patient. Formal consent for the procedure should always follow this discussion. Whether this consent is verbal or written depends on the local hospital policy.

7.5 **Premedication**

The objectives of pharmacological premedication are to reduce anxiety and produce a dry mouth. Pharmacological methods of reducing anxiety are not a substitute for the psychological preparation mentioned above. Depending on the risk, prophylaxis for aspiration is also prescribed.

7.5.1 Benzodiazepines

Benzodiazepines relieve anxiety and may produce amnesia. Any of the commonly used drugs such as temazepam or diazepam may be prescribed orally on the ward. The quick onset and short duration of the action of midazolam makes it ideal for intravenous administration in the anaesthetic room.

7.5.2 Opioids

Opioids such as morphine are not anxiolytics, but are mild sedatives and good analgesics. Intramuscular morphine, up to 10 mg for adults, 0.15 mg/kg for children, administered one hour preoperatively, will reduce the need for additional intravenous opioids during the procedure and minimize the risk of airway obstruction and respiratory depression. Opioids also aid endoscopy by suppressing the gag and the cough reflex. However they may cause nausea and vomiting and must not be administered to patients in whom there is a risk of airway obstruction.

7.5.3 Prophylaxis for aspiration

Some patients (e.g. obstetric, trauma, obese, history of reflux) undergoing awake fibreoptic intubation may be at risk of aspiration of gastric contents. A combination of a H_2 blocker (e.g. ranitidine 150 mg orally) to reduce the volume of acid in the stomach and metoclopramide 10 mg orally, a dopamine antagonist which stimulates the motility of the upper gastrointestinal tract, increases the lower oesophageal sphincter tone, and prevents vomiting, is the usual choice.

7.5.4 Antisialogogues

Antisialogogues are administered before an awake fibreoptic intubation for several reasons. A dry mouth ensures better contact between the local anaesthetic and mucosa ensuring better absorption and hence action of the local anaesthetic. Also secretions interfere with fibreoptic endoscopy; thick secretions may clog the working channel of the fibrescope; and thin secretions may cause internal reflection and distort the view.

Antimuscarinic drugs such as atropine, hyoscine and glycopyrronium are effective antisialogogues. Atropine is best avoided as it is a weak antisialogogue and may cause tachycardia. Hyoscine may be given orally (0.3 mg) or intramuscularly (0.2 mg) one hour pre operatively. It is a powerful antisialogogue and also enhances sedation and amnesia. It is best avoided in patients over 60 years of age as it may cause confusion and disorientation. Glycopyrronium is a quaternary ammonium compound and does not cross the blood brain barrier. It has a moderate antisialogogue effect and has no sedative effect. It may be given either intramuscularly (0.2 mg) or intravenously (0.2 mg), the onset of action is about 3 minutes slower after intramuscular injection.

7.6 **Monitoring**

Standard anaesthetic monitoring must be applied in the form of continuous ECG, pulse oximetry and non invasive blood pressure. A capnograph should always be available to check the position of the tube once intubation is complete.

The level of consciousness should be monitored constantly in order to obtain the desired level of conscious sedation. The goal of conscious sedation is a relaxed and calm patient who is able to respond appropriately to verbal commands or mild physical stimuli. Over sedation will lead to airway obstruction, hypoxia, and cardio respiratory depression. This may result in confusion, restlessness, and an uncooperative patient. On the other hand, under sedation and inadequate topical anaesthesia may also cause patient discomfort and restlessness.

7.7 **Oxygenation**

It is imortant to administer oxygen to the patient during the procedure. During orotracheal fibreoptic intubation, oxygen is best delivered by nasal specs. For nasotracheal fibreoptic intubation, we usually administer oxygen with an ordinary facemask while topical anaesthesia is being applied. After the nasal cavity is anaesthetized, we gently insert a suction catheter in one of the nostrils and connect it to the oxygen delivery tube. Some endoscopists prefer to deliver oxygen via the working channel of the fibrescope during endoscopy.

7.8 **Conscious sedation**

The term 'awake' intubation is a misnomer because, in practice, most patients receive some form of sedation during an 'awake' fibreoptic intubation. This is to relieve anxiety, produce amnesia, and reduce discomfort and/or pain during the procedure. Conscious Sedation (CS) is a state where the patient is calm and relaxed, can tolerate potentially unpleasant procedures, but is be able to respond to verbal commands and maintain a patent airway. It is, however, not a substitute for thorough explanation of the procedure at the preoperative visit.

The pharmacology of the drugs used for CS is discussed in Chapter 3. The following is a summary of some of the commonly used drugs in practice and tips on achieving the desired level of sedation.

7.8.1 **Boluses of midazolam and fentanyl**

Dilute midazolam to 1mg/ml and fentanyl 0.01 mg/ml. Increments of 0.5 to 1 mg of midazolam and 0.01–0.02 mg of fentanyl are then given to obtain desired level of sedation. To avoid over sedation, it is important to remember that the onset of action for midazolam and fentanyl varies from 2–5 minutes and allow the two drugs to achieve optimal effect prior to giving the next increment. Reversal drugs – naloxone and flumazenil – should be readily available.

7.8.2 Target Controlled Infusion (TCI) of propofol

Administer 1–2 mg midazolam (best avoided in elderly patients) intravenously. Start the TCI propofol at 0.001 mg/ml. Wait until the desired level of CS is achieved prior to starting topical anaesthesia of the airway. Titrate up and down by 100 ng/ml as required. If using the modern TCI infusion pumps allow for the plasma and effect site concentrations of the drug to equilibrate prior to assessing the drug effect and making further adjustments.

7.8.3 Remifentanil infusion

A practical example of the technique is to administer 0.5–2 mg of midazolam (midazolam can potentiate the respiratory depressant effects of remifentanil and should be used cautiously in conjunction with remifentanil. It is best avoided in the elderly). Start the TCI remifentanil at 3 ng/ml. Wait for the plasma and effect site concentrations to equilibrate (generally takes 3–4 minutes) before starting topical anaesthesia. Titrate up or down by 0.5 ng/ml. If using a remifentanil infusion, the equivalent would be to start at 50 ng/kg/min and titrate up or down by 10 ng/kg/min.

7.9 Upper airway local anaesthesia

Perhaps the most important component of preparation of a patient for awake fibreoptic intubation is achievement of perfect topical anaesthesia of the upper respiratory tract. A meticulous technique allows this goal to be achieved resulting in a comfortable patient who will then allow the anaesthetist to perform endoscopy and intubation in an unhurried manner. The final result is a very high success rate.

The pharmacology of the drugs used is discussed in detail in Chapter 3. There are two basic ways in which local anaesthesia of the upper airway can be achieved:

1. Direct application of local anaesthetic to the mucosa.
2. Nerve blocks.

7.9.1 Direct application techniques

Direct surface application of local anaesthetic on the mucous membranes of the respiratory tract is an easy and effective method. Nowadays, it is the most commonly used technique and is well tolerated by patients.

Some of the techiques described below are shown as pictures/video – log on www.orag.co.uk/book.

7.9.1.1 *Direct application with syringe or spray*

For example, 2% lidocaine gel to the mouth or nose; 10% lidocaine spray to the back of the tongue and oropharynx.

7.9.1.2 *Application with ribbon gauze*

A special ENT Tilley's forceps is used to pack the ribbon gauze (soaked with 2 ml of 5% cocaine or 2–4 ml of lidocaine/phenylephrine solution) into the nasal cavity.

7.9.1.3 *Cotton applicators*

Cotton applicators mounted on sticks may be used instead of the ribbon gauze described above.

7.9.1.4 *McKenzie technique*

This technique uses a cannula (e.g. 20 or 18G Venflon) connected to the oxygen bubble tubing via a three way tap to ensure a tight fit. A jet like effect of local anaesthetic is seen when it is administered from a syringe connected to the cannula while the oxygen supply is running at two litres. We this technique to anaesthetize the nasal cavity and the orophaynx.

7.9.1.5 *Mucosal Atomizer Device (MAD)*

These commercial atomizers achieve the same jet like effect and are available in different shapes and sizes.

7.9.1.6 *Spray as you go (SAYGO)*

The working channel of the fibrescope can be used to instil local anaesthetic onto the mucous membrane of the respiratory tract. The working channel of an intubating fibrescope (e.g. Olympus LF-2) is 600 mm long and 1.5 mm in diameter. If a small syringe is attached directly to the working channel port and the injection made, then it is likely to stay in the channel rather than be 'sprayed' onto the mucosa. A16 G epidural catheter is fed through the working channel (if a multi-holed catheter is used, cut the distal end). The luer lock connector of the epidural catheter gives a better grip to the syringe compared to the working channel port of the fibrescope thus avoiding leakage of local anaesthetic. Local anaesthetic is drawn up in a 2 ml syringe and 'dripped' on the mucus membrane. This is targeted better if the distal tip of the epidural catheter is allowed to protrude a cm or so from the distal tip of the fibrescope.

7.9.1.7 *Inhalation of nebulized lidocaine*

Particles larger than 100 μ will concentrate in the oral mucosa, between 60 and 100 μ will concentrate in the trachea and main bronchi and those between 30–60 μ in the larger bronchi. 4–6ml of 4% lidocaine in a nebulizer is delivered in oxygen at a flow rate of 8 litres. The technique is easy to administer, safe, non-invasive and comfortable to the patient. Coughing is absent or minimal with this technique and therefore it may be useful in patients with increased intra cranial pressure, open eye injury and unstable cervical spine injury. However we feel that local anaesthesia with this method is inadequate and additional SAYGO is required.

Our current technique of local anaesthesia for nasal fibreoptic intubation is as follows:

- Nasal cavity – McKenzie spray: 1 ml 5% cocaine to each nostril.
- Oropharynx – McKenzie spray: 4–5ml of 4% lidocaine (one ml at a time).
- Supraglottic region – SAYGO through epidural catheter: 1–2 ml 4% lidocaine.
- Glottic/infraglottic – SAYGO through epidural catheter: 1–2ml 4% lidocaine.

Local anaesthesia for oral fibreoptic intubation:

- Tongue and oropharynx: 2% lidocaine gargle + 3–4 ml 4% lidocaine with Mckenzie spray.
- Supraglottic region – SAYGO through epidural catheter: 1–2 ml 4% lidocaine.
- Glottic/infraglottic – SAYGO through epidural catheter: 1–2ml 4% lidocaine.

If gag is not obtunded then perform cricothyroid puncture with 3–4 ml of 4% lidocaine.

7.9.2 Nerve blocks

The nerve supply to the upper airway is derived from branches of the V, VII, IX, and Xth cranial nerves. In the past nerve blocks was an essential part of anaesthetizing the upper airway. This is no longer true and meticulous topical application is easier to perform, kinder to the patient, and equally effective. Moreover, in some patients it is difficult or even impossible to perform nerve blocks because of abnormal anatomy of the neck and/or upper airway. We have briefly described the glossopharyngeal and superior laryngeal nerve blocks in this chapter. The technique of injection of local anaesthetic through the cricothyroid membrane is also described.

7.9.2.1 *Glossopharyngeal nerve block*

The gag reflex arises from stimulation of deep pressure receptors found in the posterior one third of the tongue. These receptors cannot be easily reached by diffusion of local anaesthetics through the mucosa. A glossopharyngeal nerve block is useful when it is desired to completely abolish the gag reflex. The anterior approach is described below.

7.9.2.2 *Glossopharyngeal nerve block - anterior approach*

For pictures log on www.orag.co.uk/book.

- The patient sits up and the anaesthetist faces him standing on the contralateral side.
- Ask the patient to open the mouth as wide as possible and retract the tongue medially with a tongue depressor or gloved finger.
- The base of the palatoglossal (anterior) arch forms a U or J shaped band of tissue starting from the base of the palate, running along the lateral palatal wall to the lateral margin of the tongue.

- Use a 25 G spinal needle to inject 2 ml of 2% lidocaine at a point 0.5 cm from the lateral margin of the tongue at the point at which it joins the floor of the mouth (the trough of the U or J).
- Perform an aspiration test, if air is aspirated the needle is too deep, withdraw it; if blood is aspirated withdraw the needle and redirect medially.
- Perform a similar injection on the other side.

7.9.2.3 Superior laryngeal nerve block

The superior laryngeal nerve is a branch of the Vagus (X) nerve. The superior laryngeal nerve can be blocked by as many as three external and one internal (using Krause's forceps) approaches. One of the external methods is described below.

7.9.2.3.1 Technique of superior laryngeal nerve block – external approach

For pictures log on to www.orag.co.uk/book.

- The patient sits up with the anaesthetist facing him/her (on the same side of the block).
- Identify the superior cornu of the hyoid bone beneath the angle of the mandible and in front of the carotid artery. It can be palpated with the thumb and index finger on the side of the neck as bilateral rounded structures.
- Identify the superior cornu of the thyroid cartilage. It is recognized by palpating the thyroid notch (Adam's apple) and tracing the upper edge of the thyroid cartilage posteriorly when the superior cornu will be palpated as a small rounded structure lying just underneath the superior cornu of the hyoid bone on both sides.
- Using a 4 cm, 25G needle, walk along the superior cornu of the thyroid cartilage in a superior and anterior direction aiming toward the lower third of the membrane.
- When a give is felt, pierce the membrane and perform an aspiration test.
- If air is aspirated, the needle is too deep and needs to be withdrawn.
- If blood is aspirated, remove the needle and redirect it.
- Inject 2 ml of 2% lidocaine with 1:200000 adrenaline.
- Perform a similar block on the other side.

7.9.2.4 Recurrent laryngeal nerve

The sensory innervation of the vocal cords and trachea is supplied by the Vagus nerve via the recurrent laryngeal nerves. The recurrent laryngeal nerves ascend along the tracheo oesophageal groove and supply sensory fibres to the whole of the tracheobronchial tree up to and including the vocal cords and motor supply to all the intrinsic muscles of the larynx except the cricothryroid. The sensory and motor fibres run together. For this reason, recurrent laryngeal nerve blocks are not performed because this would result in bilateral vocal cord paralysis and airway obstruction. Local anaesthesia of the vocal cords is best achieved by:

7.9.2.4.1 *Translaryngeal anaesthesia (Cricothyroid puncture)*

For pictures log on to www.orag.co.uk/book.

- The patient lies supine with the neck extended and the anaesthetist standing on the side.
- Identify the inferior margin of the thyroid cartilage. The space immediately below it and between the cricoid is the cricothyroid membrane.
- Make a small wheal of local anaesthetic intradermally.
- With the thumb and third digit of one hand stabilize the trachea by holding the thryroid cartilage.
- Remove the cap of a 20G intravenous cannula (venflon, abbocath) and fix a 5 ml syringe containing 3–4 ml of 4% lidocaine to it.
- With the other hand, insert the cannula (with its tip facing caudad) and always aspirating until a give is felt and air is aspirated.
- Advance the cannula over the needle and then remove the syringe and needle from the cannula.
- Re attach the syringe to the cannula and perform aspiration again to confirm presence of cannula in the airway.
- Perform the injection at the end of normal expiration. This will ensure airway anaesthesia both below the vocal cords and up to the carina. The patient will cough during this procedure.

Studies suggest that translaryngeal anaesthesia produces least coughing during endoscopy but the most coughing during administration. It is useful in patients who are not adequately anaesthetized by direct instillation of local anaesthetic.

7.10 Good endoscopy technique

For pictures and videos of endscopy techniques in the supine and sitting position log on to www.orag.co.uk/book.

Awake fibreoptic intubation can be an unpleasant experience for both the anaesthetist and the patient if the endoscopy is not performed well. Some anaesthetists insert the tracheal tube first and then insert the fibrescope through it to access the glottis. We favour an approach where each nostril is first inspected with the fibrescope (anterior rhinoscopy), the more patent one is selected and then each aspect of the nasal or oral anatomy is identified continuously by the endoscopist, utmost care being taken not to touch the mucosa and stay in the airspace at all times. This approach reduces blood and secretions; conditions that can make an 'easy' endoscopy 'difficult'.

The position of the patient and endoscopist is also important. We prefer the patient sitting bolt upright with the endoscopist facing the patient. The upright position avoids airway obstruction, drainage of secretions is enhanced by gravity and topical anaesthesia is better tolerated by the patient. It is essential that an understanding of the airway anatomy in this position should first be learnt on anaesthetized patients with normal airways.

7.11 **Choice of tube and technique of railroading**

For pictures and video of railroading and impingement log on to www.orag.co.uk/book.

Being able to negotiate the tip of the fibrescope into the trachea is one half of the battle; the other half is being able to successfully railroad the tracheal tube into position. While endoscopy is performed under constant vision railroading of the tube into the trachea is essentially 'blind'. Railroading may be difficult or even fail as a result of impingement of the tube, most commonly at the right arytenoid cartilage. Impingement can be avoided by selecting the appropriate size and type of tube and by using the correct railroading techniques.

Smaller diameter tubes that fit snugly onto the insertion cord are generally better, the more the space between the tube and the insertion cord the higher the chance of impingement. We prefer to use tubes of sizes 6–7 mm ID for adults. The design of the tip of the tube also determines the success of railroading. The intubating LMA tube with the Huber tip is least likely to impinge. More recently the Gliderite tube with the Parker tip has also been shown to be more effective than a normal Portex tube.

The lubricated tube is inserted in the neutral position (bevel of the tube facing right) and railroaded over the fibrescope. If impingement occurs the tube is withdrawn about 1 cm, rotated 90 degrees anticlockwise (to bring the tip of the tube anteriorly) and re inserted. If this does not work than further 90 degree anticlockwise rotations are tried. We usually insert the tube in the neutral position in the nostril and turn it 90 degrees anticlockwise before it reaches the epiglottis to prevent impingement.

Other manoeuvres such as keeping the airway patent with jaw thrust and application of force on the neck may also help.

Practical tips
1. Awake fibreoptic intubation is not time consuming if you prepare drugs and equipment for conscious sedation and topical anaesthesia before the patient arrives in the anaesthetic room.
2. The fibreoptic stack needs to be facing you. Check its position in relation to the anaesthetic and monitoring equipment before you start the procedure.
3. Insert an intravenous cannula as soon as possible and administer intravenous glycopyrronium.
4. After starting the sedation monitor its effect and give it a chance to work. Remember every patient is different.
5. Before performing endoscopy ensure local anaesthesia is effective by performing gentle suction in the region of the posterior pharyngeal wall. A weak or absent gag is perfect.
6. Don't' forget to lubricate the insertion cord of the fibrescope before loading the tube.

Practical tips (Contd.)

7. The first part of the endoscopy – anterior rhinoscopy is the most important and often the most difficult. Anterior rhinoscopy allows you to identify the more patent nostril and the correct space between the inferior turbinate, floor of nose and septum of nose.

8. If you get stuck during endoscopy then withdraw the scope and start again rather than continue blindly.

9. Lubricating the tip of the tube before it is railroaded reduces patient discomfort.

10. Confirm the position of the tube in the trachea fibreoptically and also with end tidal CO_2 before giving the induction agent.

11. Do not let go of the tube until it is securely taped.

12. Good luck!

Further reading

Efthimou J, Higenbottam T, Holt D, Cochrane GM. Plasma concentrations of lidocaine during fibreoptic bronchoscopy. *Thorax* 1982; **37**: 68–71.

Kakodkar P, Lua S, Sear J, Popat M. Target controlled propofol for awake fibreoptic intubation. *Difficult Airway Society Abstracts.* Edinburgh. 1999.

Popat M. *Practical Fibreoptic Intubation.* Butterworth Heinemann. 2001.

Rai MR, Parry TM, Dombrovskis A, Warner OJ. Remifentanil target controlled infusion vs propofol target-controlled infusion for conscious sedation for awake fibreoptic intubation:a double-blinded randomized controlled trial. *Br. J .Anaesth.* 2008; **100**: 125–30.

Watanabe H, Lindgren L, Rosenberg P, Randall T. Glycopyrronium prolongs topical anaesthesia of the oral mucosa and enhances absorption of lidocaine. *Br J Anaesth* 1993; **70**: 94–5.

Chapter 8

Management of the unanticipated difficult airway: the 'can't intubate, can ventilate' scenario

Alexander Marfin and Jairaj Rangasami

Key points

- Unanticipated difficult intubation can occur despite normal airway assessment
- Maintenance of oxygenation and avoidance of airway trauma are of paramount importance
- To achieve this goal, anaesthetists must follow simple, clear, and definitive pre-existing plans such as those recommended in the Difficult Airway Society (DAS) guidelines.
- These plans are different for the 'elective' and 'rapid sequence induction' scenarios
- To execute these plans anaesthetists need to master a small number of 'alternative' techniques to direct laryngoscopy.

8.1 Introduction

Failed tracheal intubation is the primary anaesthetic cause of hypoxia, brain damage, and death. Often problems with intubation are unanticipated. When dealing with unanticipated difficulty, lack of structured approach and unfamiliarity with alternative airway management techniques can lead to repeated attempts at direct laryngoscopy resulting in airway trauma, bleeding, and further deterioration of clinical situation. Therefore management of the unanticipated difficult airway should ideally follow a simple, clear, and definitive pre-existing plan that must concentrate on oxygenation and avoidance of airway trauma.

8.2 Causes

8.2.1 Truly unanticipated difficult intubation

In this scenario, difficult/failed intubation occurs despite uneventful history and normal preoperative airway assessment. Airway assessment tests have moderate sensitivity but low specificity and a low positive predictive value (see Chapter 4). One of the possible explanations of the poor predictive value of the airway assessment lies in its inability to evaluate the epiglottic area and to predict the combined effects of general anaesthesia and supine position. An example of this problem is the presence of a supra epiglottic mass, such as hyperplasia of the lingual tonsil (for an endoscopic view of hyperplasia of lingual tonsil log on to www.orag.co.uk/book). This will prevent the epiglottis from being lifted by the Macintosh blade and hence cause difficulties in intubation.

8.2.2 Unanticipated difficult intubation where difficulties should have been predicted by preoperative assessment and the airway should have been managed as an 'anticipated' difficult airway in the first place

This scenario is unfortunately more common and analysis of such cases shows that preoperative airway assessment is either omitted or the findings are ignored. A strategy involving Macintosh laryngoscopy in the anesthetized paralysed patient is used. Repeated attempts cause airway trauma and are more likely to result in a 'can't intubate can't ventilate' situation. The possible reasons for this pattern of behaviour amongst anaesthetists are over reliance on the Macintosh technique and a lack of confidence with alternative techniques (see Chapter 1).

8.3 Management of unanticipated difficult intubation

The approach favoured by the authors is to follow the guidelines of the Difficult Airway Society (2004) for the management of the unanticipated difficult intubation in adult non obstetric patients.

8.3.1 Essential features of the DAS guidelines

- The essence of the guidelines is a series of flow charts.
- Each flow chart is for a different scenario and is based on a series of plans.
- Effective airway management depends on executing back up plans (plan B, C) when the primary technique (plan A) fails.
- Anaesthetists should make back up plans *before* performing the primary technique.

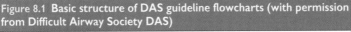

Figure 8.1 Basic structure of DAS guideline flowcharts (with permission from Difficult Airway Society DAS)

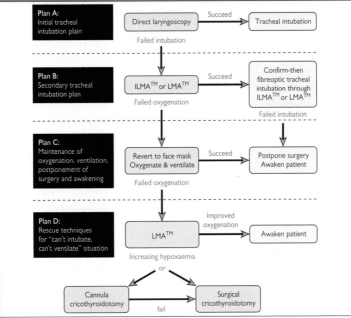

- Maintenance of *oxygenation* takes priority over everything else during the execution of each plan.
- Anaesthetists should seek the best possible assistance as soon as difficulty is recognized.
- The guidelines give an explicit duration for each plan, and include the use of well tested techniques, transferable skills, and routinely available equipment.
- The guidelines are specifically for the adult non-obstetric patient.

Management of failed intubation in obstetrics is described in Chapter 10 and of paediatric patients in Chapter 11.

The basic structure of the DAS flow charts is shown in Figure 8.1. This shows the plans, the methods of execution of each plan, and the possible outcomes.

Plan A: Initial tracheal intubation plan.

Plan B: Secondary tracheal intubation plan.

Plan C: Maintenance of oxygenation, ventilation, postponement of surgery, and awakening of the patient.

Plan D: Rescue techniques for 'can't intubate, can't ventilate' situation.

A separate flow chart has been described for each of the following scenarios:

1. Unanticipated difficult tracheal intubation during routine induction of anaesthesia in adult patient.
2. Unanticipated difficult tracheal intubation during rapid sequence induction of anaesthesia in non-obstetric patient.
3. Failed intubation, increasing hypoxaemia, and difficult ventilation in the paralysed, anaesthetized patient, the 'can't intubate, can't ventilate 'situation.

Scenario 3 is discussed in Chapter 9.

8.3.2 Scenario 1 – Unanticipated difficult tracheal intubation during routine induction of anaesthesia in adult patient

See Figure 8.2

Plan A: Initial tracheal intubation plan

The first attempt at tracheal intubation should always be performed in *optimal* conditions. This means

- after achieving adequate muscle relaxation;
- appropriate position of the head and neck (head extension and neck flexion);
- good laryngoscopy technique.
- optimum external laryngeal manipulation (OELM) or Backward, upward and rightward pressure (BURP).

The traditional 'sniffing the morning air' position can be difficult to achieve in obese patients, due to the 'buffalo hump' of fat tissues around the shoulders and neck. Reversed Trendelenberg (head-up) position can improve the intubating conditions. A head-up tilt of 15° is recommended. 'Ramping' with a specially built ramp or several thin pillows produces significantly better conditions for intubation in obese subjects. The ramp starts at the mid-interscapular level and increases in height until the occiput (for slide of optimizing head and neck position in obese patient log on to www.orag.co.uk/book) (see Chapter 10).

Optimum external laryngeal manipulation (OELM) or backward, upward and rightward pressure (BURP) on the thyroid cartilage should be an immediate response if poor laryngoscopy views are obtained. It is important to understand the difference between OELM/BURP and cricoid pressure (CP). OELM/BURP is first applied on the thyroid cartilage by the anaesthetist with his/her right hand, to achieve the best possible view and then the assistant is asked to do the same as opposed to CP, which is backward force on the cricoid cartilage applied by the assistant to prevent regurgitation. Force on the cricoid cartilage may have to be released or withdrawn if laryngoscopy is difficult.

If the measures above to optimize laryngoscopy fail and the view is still grade 3 or 4 then the following options are used:

- tracheal tube introducer (gum elastic bougie);
- alternative laryngoscope blades;
- alternative laryngoscopes.

8.3.3 Tracheal tube introducer (gum elastic bougie)

The most widely used technique in the UK is the combination of the gum elastic bougie (Venn Eschmann tracheal tube introducer) and the Macintosh laryngoscope. The advantages are simplicity of operation, low cost, ready availability and high success rate. The success rate with the original multiple use gum elastic bougie is high (94–100%) if the laryngeal view is 3a (epiglottis can be lifted off the posterior pharyngeal wall). It is of limited value when the laryngoscopy view is grade 3b (not possible to lift the epiglottis) or grade 4. The technique is blind so it should be used in the optimal way to be successful and to avoid airway trauma.

8.3.4 Practical considerations

- Perform laryngoscopy.
- Pass the prepared, lubricated bougie blindly into the trachea.
- Confirm tracheal placement by:
  1. Clicks: are felt when the bougie passes into the trachea and its tip touches the tracheal cartilages. About 60 degrees bent of the distal end of the bougie will increase occurrence of the tracheal clicks. Clicks are not elicited when the bougie goes down the centre of the tracheal lumen or is in the oesophagus.
  2. Hold up: If clicks are not present, the bougie should be advanced further, to a maximum distance of 45 cm, when resistance felt ('distal hold-up') indicates that the tip is touching the carina.
  3. Coughing: If the muscle relaxation is incomplete at this point, then coughing may also indicate tracheal placement of the bougie.
- Absence of these signs (clicks, distal hold-up, or cough) indicates that the bougie is probably in the oesophagus and another attempt at insertion is required.
- Railroading of tube:
  1. The laryngoscope must be left in the mouth to facilitate railroading.
  2. The tracheal tube is loaded over the bougie and rotated 90 degrees anticlockwise to facilitate railroading into the trachea.
  3. Further anticlockwise rotation in steps of 90 degrees may be required to overcome impingement.
  4. Other manoeuvres such as jaw thrust, cricoid pressure, and neck flexion may help.
  5. Smaller tubes, flexometallic tube, the tube supplied with the Intubating Laryngeal Mask Airway, and the GlideRite (Parker tip) tube all decrease rate of impingement in fibreoptic intubation (see Chapter 7) and may also facilitate tube insertion over the bougie.

Several studies have shown that some recently introduced single-use bougies are not as effective as the original multiple use gum elastic bougie and are also potentially more traumatic to airway.

8.3.5 **Alternative laryngoscope blades**

Alternative laryngoscope blades may be used if after the best attempt with the Macintosh blade (including longer version if required) the view is still 3 or 4. These blades should be of proven value and the choice also depends on the experience of the operator with the particular method. Many alternative laryngoscope blades are available. Two of the commonest used are the McCoy and straight blades.

8.3.6 **Alternative laryngoscopes**

Several alternative laryngoscopes have been described and their use and success in this scenario will depend on the availability of equipment and experience of the anaesthetist in using it.

1. Flexible fibreoptic laryngoscope. The oral route is preferable due to the lower risk of bleeding and can be facilitated by airway route guides such as the Berman II (for slides and video of orotracheal fibreoptic intubation through Berman airway log on to www.orag.co.uk/book) or the Ovassapian airways. Combined use of the flexible fibreoptic laryngoscope and rigid direct laryngoscope is also an option.
2. Rigid fibreoptic laryngoscopes: e.g. Bullard laryngoscope is a very popular device for the management of unanticipated difficult intubation in North America but it is not routinely available in the UK.
3. Indirect laryngoscopes with intubation channel, e.g. Airtraq Optical laryngoscopes, Pentax Airwayscope, optical stylet (e.g. Levitan, Shikani) (see Chapter 13).
4. Videolaryngoscopes e.g. Glidescope, Storz, McGrath (see Chapter 13).

Safety Rules

- Remember that all techniques are performed in the apnoeic patient.
- Adequate mask ventilation must be ensured between attempts at intubation.
- Multiple attempts with the same technique should be avoided.
- DAS guidelines recommend that the maximum number of laryngoscope insertions should be limited to four with the same direct laryngoscope not used more than twice.

Plan B: Secondary tracheal intubation plan

When the strategies used in Plan A fail, then maintaining oxygenation and ventilation both during and in between intubation attempts is a priority. This is possible by using 'dedicated airway devices' – upper airway devices, which maintain airway patency while facilitating tracheal intubation. The classic laryngeal mask airway (LMA™) and the Intubating Laryngeal mask Airway (ILMA™) are the most commonly used devices for this purpose.

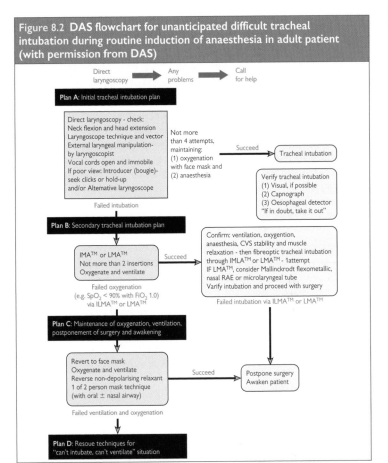

Figure 8.2 **DAS flowchart for unanticipated difficult tracheal intubation during routine induction of anaesthesia in adult patient (with permission from DAS)**

Direct laryngoscopy → Any problems → Call for help

Plan A: Initial tracheal intubation plan

Direct laryngoscopy - check:
Neck flexion and head extension
Laryngoscope technique and vector
External laryngeal manipulation-
by laryngoscopist
Vocal cords open and immobile
If poor view: Introducer (bougie)-
seek clicks or hold-up
and/or Alternative laryngoscope

Not more than 4 attempts, maintaining:
(1) oxygenation with face mask and
(2) anaesthesia

Succeed → Tracheal intubation

Verify tracheal intubation
(1) Visual, if possible
(2) Capnograph
(3) Oesophageal detector
"If in doubt, take it out"

Failed intubation

Plan B: Secondary tracheal intubation plan

IMA™ or LMA™
Not more than 2 insertions
Oxygenate and ventilate

Succeed →

Confirm: ventilation, oxygention, anaesthesia, CVS stability and muscle relaxation - then fibreoptic tracheal intubation through IMLA™ or LMA™ - 1attempt
IF LMA™, consider Mallinckrodt flexometallic, nasal RAE or microlaryngeal tube
Varify intubation and proceed with surgery

Failed oxygenation
(e.g. SpO$_2$ < 90% with FiO$_2$ 1.0)
via ILMA™ or LMA™

Failed intubation via ILMA™ or LMA™

Plan C: Maintenance of oxygenation, ventilation, postponement of surgery and awakening

Revert to face mask
Oxygenate and ventilate
Reverse non-depolarising relaxant
1 of 2 person mask technique
(with oral ± nasal airway)

Succeed →

Postpone surgery
Awaken patient

Failed ventilation and oxygenation

Plan D: Rescue techniques for "can't intubate, can't ventilate" situation

8.3.7 **The classic LMA as conduit for intubation Limitations:**

1. The LMA stem is so long (23 cm) that the cuff of an uncut standard cuffed tracheal tube (30–33 cm) may lie at the level of vocal cords, which makes it potentially traumatic and ineffective. Alternative longer tubes such as a microlaryngeal tube or nasal north polar RAE tube should be used.

2. Narrow tube connector, which only allows a 6 mm tracheal tube through a size 4 LMA and 7 mm tube through a size 5 LMA.

3. The classic LMA's aperture bars may obstruct the passage of the tracheal tube.

4. Removal of the LMA can be difficult once tracheal intubation is accomplished. The LMA should be left in place if it does not interfere with the surgical procedure.

8.3.8 **Safety rules**

- Blind intubation with classic LMA is not recommended due to the low success rate and possible airway trauma.
- Fibreoptic guided intubation using LMA as conduit is recommended (for slides of direct fibreoptic intubation through LMA log on to www.orag.co.uk/book).
- Single use laryngeal masks are different. For e.g., LMA Unique® (Intavent Orthofix) has even smaller internal diameter, which only allows a 6.5 mm ID tracheal tube through a size 5 LMA Unique®.
- Familiarize yourself with equipment in your place of work. You may try out various LMA size and tube type/size in a workshop and choose the best combinations.
- All the above problems can be overcome by using a two-stage technique with an Aintree Intubation Catheter (AIC).

8.3.9 **Aintree Intubation Catheter (AIC)**

This is a 56 cm long hollow catheter with Rapi-Fit® adapters that can connect with a 15 mm connector (for use with a Bain circuit) or Luer lock connector (for use with jet ventilator). The catheter has a 7 mm outer diameter (19.0 F) and a 4.8 mm inner diameter to allow it to be pre-loaded onto an appropriately sized fiberscope (maximum insertion cord diameter – 4.2 mm). The flexibility of the AIC allows loading over the fibrescope and its stiffness facilitates railroading of a tracheal tube.

The Aintree catheter is used for an LMA assisted orotracheal fibreoptic intubation as described:

(For slides and video of Aintree Intubation guided intubation through LMA log on to www.orag.co.uk/book).

- Insert a LMA in the usual fashion and confirm ventilation through it by connecting it to a breathing system using a 15 mm fibreoptic swivel connector.
- Guide an intubating fibrescope loaded with an AIC through the LMA bars and assess the position of the LMA.
- Advance the fibrescope tip through the larynx and into the trachea.
- Remove the fibrescope and the LMA leaving the AIC positioned in the trachea.
- Railroad a suitable size tracheal tube (minimum 7 mm ID) over the AIC.
- The same principles of railroading (described above) for the bougie apply.
- Remove the AIC and check the position of the tracheal tube with end tidal carbon dioxide.

8.3.10 **Intubating Laryngeal Mask Airway (ILMA) for secondary intubation**

The ILMA was specifically designed to overcome the limitations of the classic LMA for intubation and is the device of choice. Numerous studies have confirmed the effectiveness of the ILMA for intubation in patients with both anticipated and unanticipated difficult intubation.

The principle design features of the ILMA are:

(For slides of design features of Intubating LMA log on to www.orag.co.uk/book).

- The anatomically curved, rigid airway tube with an integral guiding handle.
- The anatomical curve permits insertion without head and neck manipulation or insertion of fingers in the mouth.
- A 15 mm connector allowing ventilation through this tube.
- The airway tube can accept tracheal tube sizes up to 8 mm.
- A 'V' shaped tracheal tube guiding ramp helps to centralize the tracheal tube and guides it anteriorly to reduce risk of arytenoid trauma and oesophageal placement.
- An epiglottic elevating bar has replaced the LMA mask bars designed to protect and elevate the epiglottis during tracheal tube passage.
- A proprietary tracheal tube is supplied with the device. This is made of silicone, is straight and reinforced and comes with a detachable 15 mm connector and a tip, with an offset distal opening, designed to avoid impingement of the tube on the vocal cords or arytenoids.
- A tracheal tube 'pusher' is also supplied with the kit for easier removal of the ILMA over the tracheal tube once intubation is complete.

The technique of blind intubation via ILMA is different from the classic LMA. An experience of about 20 insertions has been recommended to achieve an adequate level of skills. The 'Chandy manoeuvre' (alignment of the internal aperture of ILMA and the glottis by finding the degree of sagittal rotation which produces optimal ventilation, and then applying a slight anterior lift with the ILMA handle) facilitates correct positioning and blind intubation through the ILMA. Use of dedicated silicone tracheal tube is strongly recommended. The blind technique can be successful but may reuire two to three attempts and the incidence of oesophageal intubation is up to 5%. The fibreoptically guided intubation through the ILMA has a higher first attempt and overall success rates, and is nearly always successful when blind technique fails. *It is therefore the technique of choice in the unanticipated difficult intubation scenario*

There are several techniques described for fibrescope-guided tracheal tube insertion via ILMA. The technique that we currently use in Oxford is as follows: (for video of fibreoptic guided intubation through ILMA log on to www.orag.co.uk/book).

This technique protects the fibreoptic scope from potential damage that can occur if the tip is used to push up the epiglottic elevating bar. Contact with secretions resulting in a poor fibreoptic view is also avoided.

- Insert the ILMA in the recommended manner and confirm ventilation through it.
- Insert the lubricated ILMA tracheal tube in ILMA stem until its tip reaches the mask aperture as indicated by the transverse black line on the tube.

- Insert the lubricated insertion cord of the flexible fibreoptic scope through the tracheal tube so that its tip lies just within the tip of the tube.
- Advance the tube only for about 1.5 cm. Continuous fibreoptic view shows the tracheal tube tip lifting the epiglottic elevating bar, which in turn is seen to elevate the epiglottis.
- Once a clear passage has been created, advance the fibrescope into the trachea upto the carina and then railroad the tracheal tube over it.
- Check the position of the tube with the fibrescope during withdrawal and finally with end tidal carbon dioxide.

8.3.11 i-gel for fibreoptic guided intubation

The *i-gel* is a supraglottic airway with a non-inflatable cuff. It is possible to perform fibreoptic guided intubation by using the i-gel as a conduit. The i-gel has a comparatively shorter and wider stem and the lack of an inflatable cuff means more of the tracheal tube can protrude through the distal end. The maximum size of the tracheal tubes that can be passed through each size of i-gel is as follows: size 3 i-gel (6.0 mm ID), size 4 i-gel (7.0 mm ID), size 5 i-gel (8.0 mm ID). However, more practical experience and research evidence would be required to support use of i-gel in the management of the unanticipated difficult airway.

8.3.12 Safety rules

- The vocal cords should be open and non-reactive before attempting to advance the fibrescope or tracheal tube into the trachea.
- The number of attempts with any device must be limited to a maximum of two.
- It should be possible to oxygenate the patient continuously when performing the techniques.
- If intubation cannot be achieved with two attempts then a decision must be made to postpone surgery and plan C activated.

Plan C- Maintenance of oxygenation, ventilation, postponement of surgery and awakening of the patient

If intubation fails despite all the above attempts, then the safest option is to awaken the patient. Further management would depend on the nature of the difficulty and should be along the lines of the management of the patient with a known difficult intubation (Chapter 5). The option of continuing anaesthesia with the laryngeal mask although possible is not a safe option especially when intubation was initially contemplated and surgery could be postponed.

8.3.13 Scenario 2: Unanticipated difficult intubation during rapid sequence induction

Three important considerations influencing the decisions and choice of techniques suggest that this scenario should be managed in a different manner; these are:

- the increased risk of aspiration;

- the application of cricoid pressure;
- the short duration of paralysis with suxamethonium.

The principles of optimizing the initial tracheal intubation technique (Plan A), include ideal head and neck position, the use of the bougie and alternative direct laryngoscopes, are the same as during induction of anaesthesia for elective surgery. In this scenario cricoid pressure is being applied to prevent regurgitation and aspiration of gastric contents. Cricoid pressure may impair insertion of the laryngoscope, passage of the bougie and also ventilation by facemask and LMA causing airway obstruction. The force on the cricoid cartilage should be reduced, with suction at hand, if it impedes laryngoscopy. See Figure 8.3.

8.3.14 Safety rules

- Limit number of attempts at intubation to a maximum of three.
- Execute a failed intubation plan, with the aim of maintaining oxygenation and awakening the patient (Plan C) immediately.
- Do not give further doses of suxamethonium.
- Plan B is omitted in this scenario (see reasons below).

The techniques described above to execute Plan B, i.e. fibreoptic intubation through LMA/ILMA are difficult to accomplish even in experienced hands in the short duration of muscle relaxation provided by suxamethonium. There is a real risk of failure, laryngeal spasm with its consequences and airway trauma.

The only exception where a patient is not woken up after failed intubation is if that patient's life is in imminent danger from the surgical condition and it is essential to proceed with the surgery. The traditional teaching is to continue with mask ventilation and oropharyngeal airway, maintaining cricoid pressure. Continuation of anaesthesia with a classic LMA is now an established technique, although not always effective. The ProSeal LMA may prove to be a superior device in this situation as it can provide better seal and provides improved protection against aspiration. The potential advantages of ProSeal can be offset by increased complexity of insertion. Airway obstruction when using LMA or ProSeal LMA may be overcome by re-insertion, use of a smaller size, withdrawal of air from the cuff and moving the head and neck into the sniffing position. Cricoid pressure impedes positioning of and ventilation through the LMA. Therefore it may be necessary to reduce cricoid pressure during LMA or ProSeal use.

If ventilation is impossible and serious hypoxaemia is developing, the rescue plan (Plan D) for 'can't intubate can't ventilate scenario' must be implemented without delay (see Chapter 9).

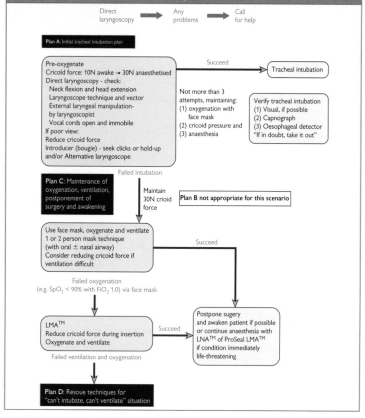

Figure 8.3 Flowchart for unanticipated difficult tracheal intubation during rapid sequence induction of anaesthesia in non-obstetric adult patient (with permission from DAS)

Direct laryngoscopy → Any problems → Call for help

Plan A: Initial tracheal intubation plan

Pre-oxygenate
Cricoid force: 10N awake → 30N anaesthetised
Direct laryngoscopy - check:
  Neck flexion and head extension
  Laryngoscope technique and vector
  External laryngeal manipulation-
  by laryngoscopist
  Vocal cords open and immobile
If poor view:
  Reduce cricoid force
  Introducer (bougie) - seek clicks or hold-up
  and/or Alternative laryngoscope

Succeed → Tracheal intubation

Not more than 3 attempts, maintaining:
(1) oxygenation with face mask
(2) cricoid pressure and
(3) anaesthesia

Verify tracheal intubation
(1) Visual, if possible
(2) Capnograph
(3) Oesophageal detector
"If in doubt, take it out"

Failed intubation

Plan C: Maintenance of oxygenation, ventilation, postponement of surgery and awakening

Maintain 30N crioid force

Plan B not appropriate for this scenario

Use face mask, oxygenate and ventilate
1 or 2 person mask technique
(with oral ± nasal airway)
Consider reducing cricoid force if
ventilation difficult

Succeed

Failed oxygenation
(e.g. SpO₂ < 90% with FiO₂ 1.0) via face mask

LMA™
Reduce cricoid force during insertion
Oxygenate and ventilate

Succeed

Postpone sugery
and awaken patient if possible
or continue anaesthesia with
LNA™ of ProSeal LMA™
if condition immediately
life-threatening

Failed ventilation and oxygenation

Plan D: Resoue techniques for
"can't intubate, can't ventilate" situation

Further reading

Charters P, O'Sullivan E. The 'dedicated airway': a review of the concept and an update of current practice. *Anaesthesia* 1999; **54**: 778–86.

Heidegger T *et al.* Validation of a Simple Algorithm for Tracheal Intubation: Daily Practice is the Key to Success in Emergencies – An Analysis of 13,248 Intubations. *Anesth Analg* 2001; **92**: 517–22.

Henderson JJ, Popat MT, Latto IP, Pearce AC: Difficult Airway Society guidelines for management of the unanticipated difficult intubation. *Anaesthesia* 2004; **59**: 675–94. www.das.uk.com/guidelines/guidelineshome.html.

Lee BJ, Kang JM and Kim DO. Laryngeal exposure during laryngoscopy is better in the 25 degree back-up position than in the supine position *British Journal of Anaesthesia* 2007; **99**: 581–6.

Ovassapian A, Glassenberg R, Randel GI, Klock A, Mesnick PS, Klafta JM. The unexpected difficult airway and lingual tonsil hyperplasia: a case series and a review of the literature. *Anesthesiology*. 2002; **97**: 124–32.

Chapter 9

Unanticipated difficult intubation: 'can't intubate, can't ventilate' (CICV) scenario

Ben Maxwell and Hamid Manji

Key points

- Predict and avoid the CICV scenario if you can
- Recognize the scenario promptly
- Don't perform a cricothyroidotomy unless you have to but do it quickly if there is no alternative
- Learn at least one method of cricothyroidotomy and practice it regularly on a manikin.

91

9.1 Introduction

A 'can't ventilate' situation is fortunately rare. If you are meticulous in your use of predictive tests for difficult intubation and/or mask ventilation (and you must be), you may only encounter a CICV emergency once in 30 or so years of elective anaesthetic theatre practice. However, such a situation is more likely in the emergency room when dealing with airway trauma and burns, and in the anaesthetic recovery area where patients may have airway oedema and blood in the pharynx.

If your pre-operative airway assessment is poor, or you fail to act on its results, you will encounter CICV more often. In the United States closed claims data reveal that over 90% of CICV were probably preventable: often the anaesthetist failed to make an adequate airway assessment before intervention, or failed to act when these tests predicted difficulty. The closed claims data also show that when conventional techniques such as direct laryngoscopy failed to achieve an airway, the anaesthetist often persisted in trying the method that had already failed and continued to fail again, rather than try something else which might have worked. It is easy to understand why this might happen during a critical incident (see Chapter 1).

9.2 Managing CICV is a core anaesthetic skill

Under most circumstances a skilled anaesthetist, using readily available equipment in a hospital setting should be able to succeed in getting oxygen into the lungs of a patient.

If you try to intubate a patient and fail an immediately life threatening circumstance exists *only* if you cannot oxygenate. The Difficult Airway Society guidelines suggest a number of strategies for the scenario of failed intubation, increasing hypoxaemia, and difficult ventilation in the paralysed anaesthetized patient (See Figure 9.1).

Make a maximum effort to achieve ventilation and oxygenation with non-invasive techniques:

1. Optimum Face mask ventilation
- You should ensure an optimal jaw thrust and head tilt/chin lift.
- A second person to help bag mask and ventilate is also helpful.
- Try inserting an oral or possibly nasal airway adjunct.
- Reduce cricoid force if necessary.
- If this does not work then call for help (if not done so already) and
  2. Try inserting a laryngeal mask airway
- Reduce cricoid force if necessary.
- Maximum two attempts.
  3. Decision
- If face mask/LMA are not effective then you are in a 'Can't intubate, can't ventilate' (CICV) scenario: worsening hypoxaemia is an indication for immediate action with an invasive technique. Do not wait till bradycardia before you act.
  4. Use a combination of an effective invasive airway device and ventilation technique.

A wide variety of equipment and techniques have been recommended. Most have a good chance of success if they are available immediately and if you are skilled enough to use them: it is too late to learn when you find yourself with a hypoxic patient you cannot ventilate.

9.3 The cricothyroid membrane

The cricothyroid membrane lies between the thyroid cartilage and the cricoid cartilage (see Chapter 3). You should make your airway here. Where time is less critical open surgical or dilational percutaneous tracheostomy is performed between the cartilaginous tracheal rings, but this site is not suitable in an

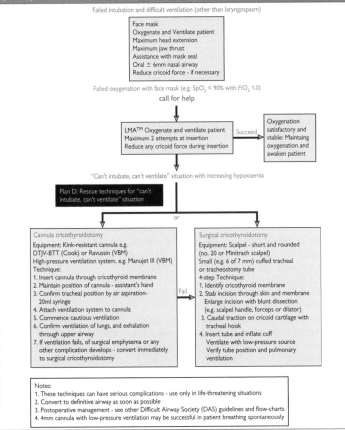

Figure 9.1 Flowchart for failed intubation, increasing hypoxaemia and difficult ventilation in the paralysed anaesthetised patient (with permission from DAS)

Failed intubation and difficult ventilation (other than laryngospasm)

Face mask
Oxygenate and Ventilate patient
Maximum head extension
Maximum jaw thrust
Assistance with mask seal
Oral ± 6mm nasal airway
Reduce cricoid force - if necessary

Failed oxygenation with face mask (e.g. SpO₂ < 90% with FiO₂ 1.0)
call for help

LMA™ Oxygenate and ventilate patient
Maximum 2 attempts at insertion
Reduce any cricoid force during insertion

Succeed → Oxygenation satisfactory and stable: Maintaining oxygenation and awaken patient

"Can't intubate, can't ventilate" situation with increasing hypoxaemia

Plan D: Rescue techniques for "can't intubate, can't ventilate" situation

or

Cannula cricothyroidotomy
Equipment: Kink-resistant cannula e.g.
DTJV-BTT (Cook) or Ravussin (VBM)
High-pressure ventilation system, e.g. Manujet III (VBM)
Technique:
1. Insert cannula through cricothyroid membrane
2. Maintain position of cannula - assistant's hand
3. Confirm tracheal position by air aspiration-20ml syringe
4. Attach ventilation system to cannula
5. Commence cautious ventilation
6. Confirm ventilation of lungs, and exhalation through upper airway
7. If ventilation fails, or surgical emphysema or any other complication develops - convert immediately to surgical cricothyroidotomy

Fail →

Surgical cricothyroidotomy
Equipment: Scalpel - short and rounded
(no. 20 or Minitrach scalpel)
Small (e.g. 6 of 7 mm) cuffed tracheal or tracheostomy tube
4-step Technique:
1. Identify cricothyroid membrane
2. Stab incision through skin and membrane
   Enlarge incision with blunt dissection
   (e.g. scalpel handle, forceps or dilator)
3. Caudal traction on cricoid cartilage with tracheal hook
4. Insert tube and inflate cuff
   Ventilate with low-pressure source
   Verify tube position and pulmonary ventilation

Notes:
1. These techniques can have serious complications - use only in life-threatening situations
2. Convert to definitive airway as soon as possible
3. Postoperative management - see other Difficult Airway Society (DAS) guidelines and flow-charts
4. 4mm cannula with low-pressure ventilation may be successful in patient breathing spontaneously

93

emergency: the trachea is too mobile, floppy and deep, with more overlying blood vessels.

In a normal individual it is easy to locate the cricothyroid membrane. Unfortunately, it is likely in CICV that your patient's anatomy will be distorted. The most likely palpable landmark is the prominent notch on the cranial aspect of the thyroid cartilage (Adam's apple). The cricothyroid membrane lies about 20 mm caudad from this point. It lies within 8 mm of the surface. From side to side it is over 20 mm across, but there is only a space 9 mm wide between the overlying cricothyroid muscles to either side. The cricothyroid membrane is crossed by a variable number of veins and occasionally arteries, most of which are small.

The space between the hyoid bone and the thyroid cartilage is easily mistaken for the cricothyroid membrane. Be careful not to make your hole here in error: you will enter the pharynx rather than the trachea, and risk damaging the vocal cords.

There are some individuals who have fixed neck deformity or large anterior neck masses in whom cricothyroidotomy would be very difficult or impossible, but this is very rare.

There are three methods of cricothyroidotomy:

9.3.1 **Surgical cricothyroidotomy**

See Figure 9.1 – for slideshow of technique log on to www.orag.co.uk/book.

Use a scalpel and a small (6 mm internal diameter), stiff, preferably cuffed, tracheal tube. A small cuffed tracheostomy tube is also acceptable.

1. If the clinical situation allows extend the neck to stretch the tissues.
2. Immobilize the larynx with your non-dominant hand.
3. Locate the cricothyroid membrane. Often it can be identified without making a skin incision: if the overlying tissue is thick make a generous cut to divide the skin in the midline over the larynx and retract the edges before feeling for the membrane. There is not usually much bleeding from the skin edges.
4. With a scalpel make a generous horizontal incision through the superior part of the cricothyroid membrane, straight into the trachea.
5. Dilate the hole into the trachea by placing the handle of your scalpel in the wound and rotating it through 90 degrees.
6. Apply caudal traction on the cricoid cartilage with a tracheal hook.
7. Insert the tracheal tube through the wound, caudad into the trachea.
8. Inflate the cuff. You may choose to verify that you are in the airway by checking that a soft suction catheter passes easily through the tube.
9. Ventilate using a bag/valve mask using a low pressure source such as a resuscitation bag or conventional anaesthesia circuit and checking with a capnometer for exhaled CO_2.
10. Sew the tube in place.
11. This is a definitive airway and can remain for several days. If an airway is required for a longer period a low tracheostomy tube should be inserted to prevent tracheal stenosis.

9.3.2 **Cannula cricothyroidotomy – narrow bore**

An alternative approach is to make a much narrower airway and use a high pressure ventilator. Although a 14 Gauge intravenous cannula has been used, and is familiar and readily available, it is a poor choice because kinking often causes it to fail. A purpose built kink-resistant catheter is preferable, such as the Jet Ventilation Cannula designed by Ravussin (VBM, Germany) which is available in sizes of 13–16G, or the 2 mm Benumof needle (Cook Critical Care). For pictures of narrow bore Ravussin cannula and the technique of insertion log on to www.orag.co.uk/book.

To oxygenate the patient through a needle less than 2 mm wide you will need a jet ventilator. This must be ready to hand and you must know how to use it.

1. If the clinical situation allows extend the neck to stretch the tissues.
2. Immobilize the larynx with your non-dominant hand.
3. Locate the cricothyroid membrane.
4. Insert the cannula over needle through the cricothyroid membrane heading caudad at about 45 degrees to the skin.
5. It is preferable to attach a syringe to the needle so that you can aspirate during insertion: air indicates that the needle tip is placed successfully in the airway.
6. Slide the cannula off the trochar.
7. Use your syringe to check again that you can aspirate air from the trachea via the cannula.
8. Connect to a jet ventilator and ventilate. Each inspiration should be just long enough to allow the chest to rise perceptibly. Each expiration must allow the air to exit fully. The Manujet 3 (VBM, Germany) is a very suitable jet ventilator: unlike a Sanders injector it is pressure limited and the set pressure is adjustable. It is relatively inexpensive.
9. As soon as possible you should replace the cricothyroidotomy cannula, inserting a definitive surgical airway to reduce the possibility of airway displacement or barotrauma.

9.3.3 Cannula cricothyroidotomy – wide bore

Instead of using a tracheostomy tube or other standard tracheal tube, a dedicated wide bore proprietary cannula (more than 4 mm) which fits a standard 15 mm connector to a resuscitation bag or anaesthetic circuit and does not require jet ventilation can be used. In the past the Minitrach (Portex) was often stocked by hospitals for this purpose: however its use is associated with a high rate of complications.

Currently the following are available:

For pictures of wide bore cricothyroidotomy cannula log on to www.orag.co.uk/book.
- Quicktrach or Quicktrach 2 (VBM, Germany);
- Portex PCK (Smiths Medical);
- Melker cricothyroidotomy kit (Cook Critical Care).

All require a smaller incision to be made in the neck compared to the surgical technique.

The Quicktrach is the simplest of these devices. It is a very sharp uncuffed cannula over trochar device. Because it is relatively short it might not reach a deep lying trachea, and may displace easily in use. Because the adult version is only 4 mm wide there has been concern that gas will escape through the pharynx if the upper airway is patent and ventilation will be inadequate to eliminate carbon dioxide using this device. Nonetheless it is simple and quick to insert. It is also inexpensive and robust, which facilitates training. Recently the device has been modified as the Quicktrach 2, by making it a little longer and adding a cuff. Unfortunately this has made the insertion technique a little more complicated.

The PCK is a robust, very blunt, cuffed 6 mm cannula inserted over a dilator and a Veress spring-loaded needle: once the trachea is entered a red indicator flag is deployed in the end of the device, reducing the chance of insertion through the posterior tracheal wall.

The Melker device uses a Seldinger technique to insert a 3–6 mm airway. A 5 mm cuffed version is usually favoured. A fine bore needle is first inserted into the trachea and then a flexible guidewire is fed through this. A dilational technique follows before the device is inserted. The technique is familiar to anaesthetists but unfortunately takes around a minute longer than using a classical surgical approach or a Quicktrach device, and has not been shown to have a higher chance of success. Training with the device is a major problem because the components are delicate.

At the time of writing it is impossible to say with certainty which is the preferred method of wide bore cricothyroidotomy. Familiarity and training with the device chosen are essential. There is insufficient experience in live humans. Studies in corpses, animal models, and dummies all have limitations. The British military forces have some experience in this area, and favour surgical cricothyroidotomy. This partly reflects the need to evacuate the patient.

The DAS guideline flow chart recommends the use of either a cannula or surgical cricothyroidotomy (Figure 9.1)

9.4 **Complications**

There are complications of cannula insertion in over 20% of reported cricothyrotomies; these prevent ventilation or threaten life in less than 5%. These risks must be balanced against likely hypoxic brain damage or death from failure to ventilate.

A degree of haemorrhage is likely, especially with a wide bore airway. If bleeding occurs the quickest way to control it is probably to complete the insertion of the cannula and thus tamponade the vessel.

Many complications are caused by failure to insert the cannula in the correct place: if it is inserted too high ventilation may be impossible and the vocal cords may be damaged. If it is inserted too low a more bloody and difficult insertion will follow. Going too deep and transfixing the trachea may damage the oesophagus, which lies posteriorly. Missing the trachea altogether creates a false passage and will prevent ventilation. Surgical emphysema, the release of air into the neck, is then a real danger, since it will tend to obscure the landmarks for a repeat attempt. Especially if using a jet ventilator it is important to ensure that the cannula lies within the trachea before starting to ventilate.

Other complications include damage to the tracheal cartilages and barotrauma, pneumothorax, and pneumomediastinum, particularly when jet ventilation is used.

9.5 Wide bore or narrow bore cannula?

9.5.1 Advantages of a narrow bore and jet ventilator technique

Unlike wide bore cricothyroidotomy, the narrow bore technique may have a role outside the CICV situation, because only a small hole is left in the neck. You might use this method electively to facilitate anaesthesia, for instance in laryngeal surgery: you should be aware that a fatal haemorrhage has once occurred following needle cricothyroidotomy. The technique may also be useful as a fall-back when managing an anticipated difficult airway: for instance during some fibreoptic intubations it may be helpful to mark the cricothyroid membrane and prepare the jet ventilator as a Plan B if your first-line management fails (see Chapters 5 and 6). Thus you may be able to perfect your technique before you face the CICV situation.

A second advantage is that you may be less hesitant to make a small hole in the neck and so may begin cricothyroidotomy relatively earlier, before your patient is irretrievable.

In a child a narrow bore cricothyroidotomy is preferable, because injury to the cricoid cartilage is less likely to occur. Such damage can lead to long-term problems with airway stenosis. In addition the cricothyroid membrane is particularly vascular in children. Barotrauma is also more likely in a child, so jet ventilation must be undertaken with exceptional care.

9.5.2 Disadvantages of a narrow bore and jet ventilator technique

A narrow bore (less than 4 mm) cannula will require a jet ventilator to maintain oxygenation. Unless one is to hand and you know how to use it a narrow bore cricothyroidotomy is pointless. In addition a narrow bore cannula is uncuffed and so is less protected against aspiration of stomach contents, though the pressure gradient may provide a degree of protection. Tracheal contents cannot be suctioned out through a narrow bore airway.

Jet ventilation may lead more easily to airway trauma and pneumothorax. A narrow bore airway may kink or become displaced, particularly as high pressure may cause the cannula tip to whip around. Such an airway is clearly unsuitable for anything but short term use, and is inappropriate during patient transfer.

In addition complete upper airway occlusion is a contraindication to narrow bore cricothyroidotomy because gas cannot pass rapidly enough through the cricothyroidotomy cannula to allow expiration: the patient has to breathe out through the upper airway. In CICV the patient's larynx and upper airway will usually allow egress of gas under pressure, but if the airway is completely occluded, for instance by a foreign body, a wide bore cannula is essential.

9.6 **Practice makes perfect**

Studies have clearly shown that practice in manikins and, where possible in animals, makes cricothyroidotomy faster and reduces complications. The techniques are easy in theory but difficult under the stress of CICV. Skill retention is short and the technique should be practised every few months for optimal performance.

Make sure that you have equipment available for cricothyroidotomy in all areas where you may encounter airway obstruction, that you have trained to use it, and keep your skills refreshed.

Further reading

Frerk C, Frampton C. Cricothyroidotomy; time for change. *Anaesthesia.* 2006; **61**: 921–3.

Henderson JJ, Popat MT, Latto IP, Pearce AC: Difficult Airway Society guidelines for management of the unanticipated difficult intubation. *Anaesthesia* 2004; **59**: 675–94. http://www.das.uk.com/guidelines/guidelineshome.html.

Vadodaria BS, Gandhi SD, McIndoe AK. Comparison of four different emergency airway access equipment sets on a human patient simulator. *Anaesthesia.* 2004; **59**: 73–9.

Vanner R Emergency cricothyroidotomy (review). *Current Anaesthesia and Critical Care* 2001; **12**: 238–43.

Wong DT, Kumar A, Prabhu A. The laryngeal mask airway prevents supraglottic leak during ventilation through an uncuffed cricothyroidotomy. *Can J Anaesth.* 2007; **54**: 151–4.

Chapter 10

Difficult airway in special situations

Jenny Thompson

10.1 Special situations

- Obstetric anaesthesia.
- Obesity.
- Major trauma and emergency room.

> **Key points**
> - Incidence of difficult/failed intubation is higher in the obstetric population
> - Planning of women with anticipated difficult airway involving teamwork between anaesthetists, obstetricians, and midwives ensures safe outcome
> - Anaesthetists should be prepared for the unanticipated difficult airway in obstetrics at all times by having pre formulated plans
> - The pre formulated plans may include the decision to awaken the patient after failed intubation.

10.2 Difficult airway in obstetric anaesthesia

10.2.1 Why is the obstetric airway challenging?

Difficult or failed intubation following induction of anaesthesia for caesarean section remains not only a source of fear among trainee anaesthetists but is also a major contributory factor to anaesthesia related maternal mortality both in the United Kingdom and the United States of America. Although it has been recently argued that the obstetric airway is no different than any other, failed intubation occurs as frequently as 1:260 parturients in some studies (compared to about 1:2000 in general population). The reasons include anatomical/physiological changes in pregnancy and organizational issues.

10.3 Anatomical/physiological changes

10.3.1 Increased total body water due to progesterone

Swelling in the nasal cavity, pharynx, larynx, and trachea result from vascular engorgement of the respiratory tract. This can lead to a number of potential problems for the anaesthetist including increased risk of bleeding from nasal instrumentation, increase in Mallampati score making direct laryngoscopy difficult; laryngeal and tracheal oedema may necessitate the use of a smaller diameter tracheal tube.

10.3.2 Weight gain

* Increased thoracic diameter and enlarged breasts make laryngoscopy awkward.
* Obesity with all it's risks (see below).

10.3.3 Mechanical effects from the gravid uterus

* Progressive decrease in expiratory reserve volume (ERV), residual volume (RV) and functional residual capacity (FRC).
* These changes are exaggerated in the supine or Trendelenberg position, where the FRC may fall below the closing capacity leading to airway closure, increased dead space, and arterio-venous shunting.
* Increased maternal oxygen consumption occurs as a result of increased maternal metabolic requirements combined with the metabolic needs of the foetus.

10.3.4 Increased gastric acid volume and acidity

* Hormonal and gastro oesophageal sphincter insufficiency (this is also exacerbated by the mechanical effects of the increased intra-abdominal pressure).
* Gastric emptying is delayed during labour as a response to pain, hormonal effects and opioid drugs.
* For these reasons pregnant women must be assumed to have a 'full stomach'.

10.4 Organizational factors

Difficult/failed intubation in obstetrics is more common during emergency surgery. Emergency general anaesthesia in the UK is mainly delivered by trainee anaesthetists. Trainee anaesthetists lack experience in general anaesthesia for obstetrics.

* Number of general anaesthetics decreasing despite increase in number of caesarean sections.
* Number performed by trainees is falling.
* Number performed for training is even lower.

Obstetric general anaesthesia in emergency is stressful – consideration for foetal well being should anything happen to the mother. Lack of experience/ training leads to unacceptable risky behaviour. Data from audits suggest:

- Lack of pre operative assessment.
- Lack of appropriate action even when difficulties identified.
- Inadequate monitoring, e.g. not using capnography to check tube placement.
- Protocol violation, e.g. giving second dose of suxamethonium.
- Inadequate follow up.

10.5 Preoperative assessment

- Obstetric patients may demonstrate any of the signs, symptoms and pathologies associated with potential difficult airway in non-pregnant patients as discussed in Chapters 5 and 6. For pictures of obstetric patients with anticipated difficult airways log on to www.orag.co.uk/book.
- The obstetric population is also changing as a result of increasing fertility interventions, increasing maternal age, obesity, comorbidities and patient expectation.
- The factors peculiar to obstetrics are as discussed above.
- Anaesthetic pre assessment during antenatal period enables the anaesthetist to make appropriate plans for safe airway management.
- These plans may include multidisciplinary discussions regarding the safest mode and timing of delivery and appropriate equipment availability.
- Occasionally the anaesthetic team may need to alert the obstetricians, that due to the nature of the patient's condition, it would not be possible to guarantee anaesthesia for a category 1 caesarean section (i.e. delivery of foetus within 30 minutes of the decision to deliver).
- Pre assessment requires not only excellent communication between midwifery, obstetric, and anaesthetic staff but also guidelines for non-anaesthetic staff to allow the identification of appropriate patients to be referred to the anaesthetic team for assessment.
- Inevitably some patients will fall through the pre-assessment net and the duty anaesthetist must be alert to potential unforeseen problems.

As a minimum, even in an emergency, the anaesthetist would be wise to ascertain details of any problems with previous anaesthetics, and assess the airway using the Mallampati test, mandibular subluxation and thyromental distance. If two out of these predict difficulty then expect trouble with Macintosh laryngoscopy and be prepared (chapter 4). Body habitus is also important.

10.6 **Managing obstetric difficult airway**

10.6.1 **Anticipated obstetric difficult airway**

Depending on the nature and severity of the problem it will not infrequently be decided to deliver these women by elective caesarean section allowing the time, type of anaesthetic, and personnel required to be planned in advance. It must, however, be remembered that these patients may arrive unannounced as emergency cases and the plans must take this into account. Details of the management principles of patients with anticipated difficult airway are described in Chapters 5 and 6.

10.6.1.1 *Plan A: regional anaesthesia unless contraindicated*

The choice of the regional anaesthetic technique, i.e. combined spinal epidural, single shot spinal or epidural anaesthesia depends on the experience and preference of the anaesthetist. The author favours combined spinal epidural anaesthesia for the following reasons:

- It is her usual technique.
- The epidural needle is a good introducer for the spinal needle.
- If spinal block fails or is inadequate then the epidural can be topped up to provide anaesthesia.

For pictures of an obstetric patient with anticipated difficult airway managed with CSE log on to www.orag.co.uk/book.

10.6.1.2 *Plan B: worked out in advance should regional anaestheisa fails or is inadequate*

This would usually include securing the airway by tracheal intubation. The anaesthetist must be experienced in performing the airway management technique for this plan B.

For pictures and video of patient in whom regional anaesthesia failed (plan A) and who was managed with Awake fibreoptic intubation log on to www.orag.co.uk/book.

10.6.2 **General anaesthesia**

General anaesthesia may be the anaesthetic of choice in patients in whom regional anaesthesia is contraindicated, or is refused. It may also be required if regional anaesthesia fails (see plan B above).

Awake fibreoptic intubation followed by induction of anaesthesia is the technique of choice although awake direct laryngoscopy, general anaesthesia using the intubating laryngeal mask airway (ILMA), the Bullard laryngoscope, retrograde intubation, and other intubating equipment have all been described.

10.6.3 **Awake fibreoptic intubation in the obstetric patient**

The principles outlined in Chapter 7 to make awake fibreoptic intubation successful all apply but there are some specific considerations for the obstetric patient

1. **Sitting position.** Performing the technique in the *sitting* position reduces the risk of regurgitation by gravity and also avoids airway obstruction and aortocaval occlusion.
2. **Oral route.** The oral route for fibreoptic intubation is safest because engorgement of the nasal mucosa means that nasal haemorrhage is a predictable and potentially catastrophic sequlae of nasal fibreoptic endoscopy.
3. **Cocaine** should not be used for mucosal topical anaesthesia in the pregnant patient, as it is associated with decreased perfusion across the placenta, hypertensive crisis, and placental abruption.
4. **Conscious sedation.** Sedation such as midazolam and/or a low dose propofol infusion may be helpful, but be aware of placental transfer and alert neonatologists as appropriate.
5. It is over sedation rather than the technique of local anaesthesia of the upper airway that makes the larynx incompetent and increases the likelihood of regurgitation.

10.6.4 **Unanticipated difficult intubation**

- The nature of obstetric anaesthesia is such that a significant proportion of the difficult airways will first be recognized at the time of attempted intubation.
- Obstetric anaesthetic departments should run regular failed intubation drills to familiarize staff and ideally these should be multidisciplinary to allow non-anaesthetists insight into the nature and potential sequelae of failed intubation.
- During every obstetric general anaesthetic, the anaesthetist must have the failed intubation drill in their mind.

10.6.4.1 *Preoperative assessment*

A history from the patient of any previous anaesthetic problems and airway assessment to include Mallampati test, mandibular subluxation, and thyromental distance should be a minimum requirement.

10.6.4.2 *Planning*

Remember that your assistant will be applying cricoid pressure and will not be able to hand equipment to you. For this reason you should get the following ready at the beginning of your shift:

- short handle laryngoscope, McCoy laryngoscope (if it is included in the plan for failed intubation);
- gum elastic bougie (checked and ready to use, lubricated before case);
- laryngeal mask airway(s) ready and checked;
- assortment of tubes, oral and nasal airways;
- knowledge of where the equipment for cricothyroid puncture and jet ventilation is and how to work it;
- check the anaesthetic machine and monitoring equipment;

- skilled anaesthetic assistant plus experienced second anaesthetist if the patient is morbidly obese;
- awareness of how to contact senior anaesthetic help if required.

10.6.4.3 *Conduct of anaesthesia and intubation (procedures)*

The sequence of events is similar to the scenario of Plan A – initial tracheal intubation plan of the DAS algorithm for rapid sequence induction (Chapter 8). In summary:

- The patient should be appropriately positioned *prior* to pre-oxygenation, this is especially important for the morbidly obese patient who will require some time to position and once induced will be too heavy to reposition!
- Always pre-oxygenate 3–5 minutes of 100% oxygen or eight vital capacity breaths over 60 seconds.
- Perform rapid sequence induction of anaesthesia with appropriate dose of thiopental and suxamethonium.
- Perform direct laryngoscopy using a short handle laryngoscope (1st attempt)
- If view of the larynx is poor then keep the laryngoscope in the mouth and consider Optimal External Laryngeal Manipulation or BURP (**B**ackwards **U**pwards and **R**ightwards **P**ressure). Remember to perform these with your right hand first and then ask the assistant to do the same. Cricoid force may have to be released to do this (Chapter 8).
- Attempt to place a gum elastic bougie (2nd attempt) (see Chapter 8 for technique).
- If the bougie fails use a different laryngoscope of your choice (3rd attempt)

These procedures should be regarded, as a ONE WAY STREET and once attempted should not be returned to. *Patients die from lack of ventilation not lack of intubation.* The DECISION now is that intubation has failed and the priority is oxygenation of the patient's lungs. **Call for help if not already done so**.

If intubation has failed, ventilation must be optimized using the following:
- One handed mask technique.
- If not successful try with the aid of oro pharyngeal airway adjunct.
- If not successful try two handed mask technique.
- If not successful attempt LMA placement (remove cricoid pressure transiently while inserting).

10.6.4.4 *What to do if ventilation is SUCCESSFUL with either facemask or laryngeal mask airway?*

- First do no harm!
- If facemask ventilation is successful do not proceed to LMA insertion, as there is no guarantee this will succeed.

- If the mother's life is in danger (e.g. major haemorrhage or anaphylaxis) continue anaesthesia, allowing the patient to breath spontaneously with a deep volatile anaesthetic.
- If the mother's life is not in danger but that of the foetus may be, a judgement decision must be made. The mother's life should not be put in jeopardy to save that of the foetus, so if the airway were precarious it would be safest for the mother to be woken up. If however a senior anaesthetist present who feels confident that the facemask or LM airway is secure, may make the decision to proceed with delivery of the baby. *It should be remembered that once the caesarean section is commenced, the option to wake the mother up is no longer viable.* It would help if this decision process 'to wake up or not' is made by the obstetric and anaesthetic team for every category 1 caesarean section *prior* to induction of anaesthesia.
- If the mother is woken prior to delivery of the baby, once the mother is safe other anaesthetic options for foetal delivery can be considered such as regional anaesthesia, local infiltration (rarely practiced in the developed world) or awake intubation.

10.6.4.5 *What to do if ventilation is NOT SUCCESSFUL with either facemask or laryngeal mask airway?*

- You will need to make this decision fast.
- Activate 'can't intubate, can't ventilate' scenario plan.
- Use a cannula cricothyroidotomy that you are used to with a jet ventilation device See chapter 9 for details of technique.

Further reading

Cooper GM, McClure JH. Anaesthesia chapter from Saving Mothers' Lives; reviewing maternal deaths to make pregnancy safer. *British Journal Of Anaesthesia* 2008; **100**: 17–22.

Clyburn PA. Early thoughts on 'Why Mothers Die 2000-2002'. *Anaesthesia* 2004; **59**: 1155–9.

Russell R. Failed intubation in obstetrics: a self fulfilling prophecy? *International Journal of Obstetric Anesthesia* 2007; **16**: 1–3.

Stacey M. Failed intubation in obstetrics. Anaesthesia and Intensive Care Medicine. 2007; **8**: 8 305–308.

10.7 **Obesity and airway management**

Key points

- All aspects of airway management in the obese patient are challenging
- Standard history and predictive tests may fail to anticipate airway difficulty
- The presence of obstructive sleep apnoea is highly suggestive of airway difficulties
- Spontaneous breathing is not an option and intubation is mandatory to avoid airway obstruction and hypoventilation
- Awake intubation provides a safer alternative to intubation under general anaesthesia
- Planning for general anaesthesia should include induction in operating theatre with adequate personnel and readiness to deal with unanticipated difficulties. It is desirable for two anaesthetists to be present
- Airway problems may continue after extubation and into the post operative period
- There is no place for 'deep' extubation and the choice is between 'awake' extubation and post operative ventilation.

10.7.1 **Incidence and definition**

The incidence of obesity is increasing in the developed world: an estimated 7% of the world's adult population (250 million people) are thought to obese. In the UK 43% men and 33% women are overweight; 22% men and 33% women are obese. It is estimated that around 30,000 deaths annually in the UK are as a result of obesity. Body Mass Index is widely used to define obesity but waist circumference is more predictive of morbidity.

BMI (kg/meter sq)	Descriptor
20–24.9	Ideal
25–29.9	Overweight
30–39.9	Obese
40–49.9	Morbidly obese
(35–49.9 with comorbidity)	
50–59.9	Super obese
60–69.9	Super super obese

10.8 Why is the airway challenging in obesity?

10.8.1 Anatomical difficulties

Intubation gets more difficult with increasing body mass index; 24 % of obese patients in a recent series, 8 % requiring awake intubation. Fatty infiltration of the wall of the pharynx with increased compliance can result in airway obstruction, difficult face mask ventilation and tracheal intubation. Short thick neck – awkward positioning for direct laryngoscopy.

10.8.2 Pathophysiological factors and presence of co morbidity

Reduced FRC and intrapulmonary shunt – may result in rapid and profound arterial desaturation especially in the supine position. This may be made worse by airway obstruction due to pharyngeal narrowing. Therefore spontaneous ventilation during anaesthesia even for short procedures is not an option and intubation is mandatory.

Obesity is associated with many co morbidities which may themselves contribute directly to difficulties in airway management or indirectly contribute to morbidity by exaggerating the consequences of airway obstruction and the resultant hypoventilation. Examples of the former include obstructive sleep apnoea, obesity hypoventilation syndrome, presence of hiatus hernia, diabetes, and arthritis of the neck.. Examples of the latter include hypertension, ischemic heart disease, cor pulmonare, cardiomyopathy, and supine hypotensive syndrome.

10.8.3 Practical difficulties

The logistical difficulties of dealing with an obese patient can contribute to difficulties with airway management either directly or indirectly. These factors include operating table size, monitoring equipment, venous access, availability of sufficient personnel to help with lifting/turning patient on side.

10.9 Airway management

Safe and effective airway management of the obese patient relies on many of the principles already discussed for any other potentially difficult airway patient (Chapters 2 and 5). Some important considerations are as follows.

10.9.1 Pre-assessment and planning

The preoperative assessment should be ideally conducted by an anaesthetist experienced in anaesthesia for obese patients and well in advance of the scheduled date of surgery. Pre operative assessment should include history, physical examination and in some cases specific investigations such as lateral cephalometry and sleep studies. Patients who give a history of obstructive sleep apnoea are at increased risk of both mask and intubation difficulties. In extreme cases patients snore while awake and pause to draw breath during normal speech.

Standard predictors of difficult intubation may not predict airway difficulties in the obese patient. Patients with a large neck circumference should arouse suspicion. Where indicated arterial blood gases and lateral cephalometry (to define the extent to which soft tissue collapse obstructs the airway) should be performed.

A clear individual plan should be made for the conduct of anaesthesia in general and of airway management in particular. This should include decisions about the primary plan (plan A) to secure the airway and at least one back up plan (plan B) should plan A fail. The consideration of awake intubation to execute plan A is strongly recommended. The need for two anaesthetists is strongly suggested.

10.9.2 General planning

The concept of having a dedicated operating theatre (obesity theatre) and a dedicated 'obesity team' to manage obese patients is well established. Having a dedicated 'obesity pack' ensures that appropriate equipment including difficult airway equipment is readily available even in an emergency. The dedicated teams should have enough personnel to move the patient and also experienced medical personnel. It is widely accepted that two anaesthetists should manage these patients.

10.9.3 Procedure – conduct of anaesthesia

Regional anaesthesia is preferred in obstetrics. An early working epidural in labour allows emergency caesarean section to be performed under regional anaesthesia and avoid the hazards of intubation.

Awake fibreoptic intubation may be indicated in some patients. The principles are discussed in Chapter 7.

The following is a summary of the principles of airway management in the obese patient having a general anaesthetic:

- Anaesthesia should be induced in the operating room and not anaesthetic room.
- Ensure adequate monitoring is in place and working.
- Appropriate personnel available to move the patient should this be required.
- Equipment to deal with both plan A and plan B is readily available.

The goal is to *optimize* direct laryngoscopy and aim for first pass success by paying attention to following:

10.9.3.1 *Patient positioning*

10.9.3.1.1 *Head up*

To avoid basal airway collapse and intubation difficulties with supine position. Although a tilt of 25 degrees has been quoted in the literature, 15 degrees is more practicable.

10.9.3.1.2 *Ramping*

This is used instead of the traditional 'sniffing the morning air' intubating position. The ramp is built with a thin pillow and graduated layers of blanket or a custom made ramp. The ramp starts at the mid inter-scapular position and increases in depth until the occiput. The aim of the positioning is to bring the external auditory meatus and the manubrium sternum into a horizontal plane.

For pictures of the optimum positioning of an obese patient by ramping log on to www.orag.co.uk/book.

10.9.3.2 **Pre oxygenation**

Should be performed with a tight fitting face mask and high flow oxygen to minimize air entrainment. A rough estimate of the arterial carbon dioxide partial pressure can be made from the end tidal carbon dioxide measurement (if sampling has not been done with arterial line). The application of CPAP (6 cm H_2O) for five minutes in conscious patients improves oxygenation.

10.9.3.3 **Induction of anaesthesia**

This is as for routine induction or rapid sequence if needed. Adequacy of face mask ventilation is ensured before injection of muscle relaxant. Face mask ventilation may require a two person/four handed technique.

10.9.3.4 **Intubation**

A short handle laryngoscope blade or polio blade is useful. Use of OELM/BURP and a gum elastic bougie is a most useful adjunct. Other laryngoscopes of particular value are the Bullard scope and more recently the Airtraq optical laryngoscope (see Chapter 13). These should only be used by anaesthetists experienced in using these devices routinely.

10.9.4 **If plan A fails, plan B should be executed**

Rescue ventilation with a supraglottic device is appropriate. The intubating LMA is particularly useful and can allow fibreoptic guided intubation once placement is confirmed (see Chapter 8).

10.9.5 **Extubation**

The obese patient is at risk of hypoxia and loss of airway control following extubation. There is no place for extubation of the trachea in the anesthetized patient and the choice is between extubation when fully awake and post operative ventilation. Extubation in the fully awake patient, sitting up has additional advantages. If the patient was on CPAP this should be instituted straight away.

10.10 **Difficult airway in the emergency room (major trauma)**

Key points

- The trauma patient may require airway control urgently in the emergency room as part of the initial resuscitation or electively in the operating theatre
- Airway management strategies in the emergency room are different to that in the elective environment of the operating theatre
- In the emergency room, the real risks of hypoxia and its consequences far outweigh the small risks of failed intubation
- For this reason performing rapid sequence induction with an optimum direct laryngoscopy technique is the technique of choice unless contraindicated
- Manual inline neck stabilization (MILNS) is used during laryngoscopy to prevent damage to the cervical spinal cord
- A clear plan of rescue ventilation should be in place should a failed intubation occur.

10.11 **Introduction**

The trauma patient may require airway management urgently in the emergency room or more electively in the operating theatre for definitive surgery. This chapter only deals with aspects of airway management in the emergency room. The principles of difficult airway management for the more elective scenario in the operating theatre are similar to any other scenarios and are discussed elsewhere (Chapters 5, 6, 8).

There is an urgent need to provide oxygen and protect the lungs from aspiration and prevent secondary central nervous system damage. Airway control allows diagnostic studies to be performed. The trauma patient is treated according to the ATLS (Advanced Trauma and Life Support) mantra, 'Airway with cervical-spine (c-spine) control, Breathing and Circulation'. The intention being that swift appropriately directed therapy should not only save lives but also prevent secondary injuries from hypoxia, hypercarbia, hypotension, and worsening of primary injuries.

10.12 **Pre assessment**

The emergency department is a different environment to the operating theatres.

There can be difficulty with pre assessment due to patient cooperation and inability to move the neck. Hard collars limit mouth opening, jaw thrust, cricoid pressure, laryngeal manipulation, and LMA insertion and increase the proportion of C&L grade 3 & 4 views. The incidence of difficult intubation after RSI in the emergency department is estimated at 10%.

10.13 **Planning**

Some of the management options used in the operating room such as awakening the patient if intubation fails or cancelling surgery are not relevant to the emergency setting. Techniques such as awake fibreoptic intubation generally do not work in the emergency setting because of blood, secretions, vomitus, and patients are frequently hypoxic and agitated. The real risks of hypoxia and its consequences outweigh the small risk of failed intubation. For this reason the goal is to secure a definitive airway without delay. This is best achieved by performing a rapid sequence induction technique unless this is contraindicated (see below). Planning should include measures to limit damage to the spinal cord (see MILS – below).

The aim should be to achieve a high first pass success by optimising the first direct laryngoscopy attempt (plan A – see Chapter 8). A plan B should be worked out in advance and may include rescue ventilation with a supraglottic device or a surgical airway.

Rapid sequence induction may not be appropriate in the following:

- Cranio-facial injuries – disruption to soft tissues and /or bony structures may distort the normal anatomy making oral intubation difficult, blood and other secretions can limit views and swelling, tissue disruption or oedema may hinder ventilation and precipitate hypoxia . The option is to perform awake nasal intubation or surgical airway.
- Laryngeal/tracheal disruption. A surgical airway is required.
- Burns – may result in airway oedema and/or airway burns leading to difficult intubation and ventilation. Circumferential burns to neck and/or chest will hinder ventilation. Carbon monoxide poisoning will lead to poor oxygenation.
- Unresponsive patients – intubation may be performed without administering anaesthetic and muscle relaxants.

10.14 **Conduct of anaesthesia and intubation**

10.14.1 **Pre oxygenation**
With high flow oxygen device. May be difficult because of poor mask seal, agitation, facial trauma, airway obstruction.

10.14.2 **MILS (Manual in – line stabilization)**
Is applied by an assistant crouched beside the intubator. This involves holding the patient's mastoid processes firmly down on the trolley. MILS should

oppose the force generated by direct laryngoscopy and is not traction on the spine. Remove hard collar.

10.14.3 Cricoid pressure

(10 N) to start with. Two handed cricoid pressure may give better views at laryngoscopy while leading to less neck movement. CP may be difficult to apply in presence of surgical emphysema/laryngotracheal injury, and may make laryngoscopy difficult.

10.14.4 Intravenous induction

With pre determined dose of induction agent and increase cricioid pressure to 30 N. Inject appropriate dose of suxamethonium and attempt intubation after full muscle paralysis.

10.14.5 Optimize first attempt at laryngoscopy

- McCoy blade – during MILS and cricoid pressure the view with a McCoy blade will be equivalent to or better than with the same size Macintosh blade.
- OELM/BURP are useful.
- Gum elastic bougie – facilitates intubation with potentially less force being exerted at direct laryngoscopy.
- Use small tube, preferably one that railroads easily.

10.14.6 Other techniques

- Other techniques which allow good laryngeal views with minimal neck movement include flexible fibreoptic scope, Bullard type scope, Airtraq Indirect laryngoscope.
- These should only be used by anaesthetists experienced in their use.

Limit the number of intubation attempts to three

10.15 Difficult/failed intubation

If a difficult laryngoscopy/intubation occurs despite optimized laryngoscopy then institute a failed intubation drill:

- Call for appropriate help – one more attempt by an experienced operator is acceptable.
- Remember that awakening is not an option.
- Aim to use techniques to rescue ventilation (see below) without delay
- A supraglottic device such as laryngeal mask airway is most appropriate. A Proseal or LMA Supreme may confer added advantages by providing a higher seal pressure and allowing a gastric tube to be passed (see Chapter 13). The devices all allow the head to remain in the neutral position during insertion. Both LMA and ILMA can be used to ventilate the patient and as conduits for tracheal intubation either blindly or with the aid of the fibreoptic scope.
- If difficulty is with insertion of laryngoscope – do not waste time – a surgical airway (cricothyroidotomy or tracheotomy) should be facilitated immediately.

Further reading

Benumof JL. Obstructive sleep apnoe in the adult obese patient: implications for airway management. *Journal of Clinical Anaesthesia* 2001; **13**: 144–56.

Casati A, Putzu M. Anesthesia in the obese patient: pharmacokinetic considerations. *Journal of Clinical Anesthesia* 2005; **17**: 134–45.

Cheah MH, Kam PC. Obesity: basic science and medical aspects relevant to anaesthetists. *Anaesthesia* 2005; **60**: 1009–21.

Cranshaw J, Nolan J. Airway management after major trauma. *Continuing Education in Anaesthesia, Critical Care & Pain* 2006; **6**: 124–27.

Crosby E. Airway management in adults after cervical spine injury. *Anaesthesiology* 2006; **104**: 1293–98.

Levitan RM. The Airway Cam guide to intubation and practical emergency airway management. Airway Cam Technologies, Inc. Pennsylvania. www.airwaycam.com.

Manoach S, Paladino L. Manual In-Line Stabilization for Acute Airway Management of Suspected Cervical Spine Injury: Historical Review and Current Questions. *Annals of Emergency Medicine* 2007; **50**: 236–45.

McLeod ADM, Calder I. Spinal cord injury and direct laryngoscopy – the legend lives on. *Br J Anaesth* 2000; **84**: 705–8.

Obesity guideline. London: Association of Anaesthetists of Great Britain and Ireland, (2007). http://www.aagbi.org/publications/guidelines.htm.

Saravanakumar K, Rao SG, Cooper GM. Obesity and obstetric anaesthesia. *Anaesthesia* 2006; **61**: 36–48.

Soens MA, Birnbach DJ, Ranainghe JS, Van Zundert A. Obstetric anaesthesia for the obese and morbidly obese patient: an ounce of prevention is worth more than a pound of treatment. *Acta Anaesthesiologica Scandinavica* 2008; **52**: 6–19.

Chapter 11

Management of paediatric difficult airway

David Mason and Sara McDouall

Key points

- Major airway difficulties are rare in paediatric anaesthesia and are usually predictable
- A history from parents and previous documentation provides the best clues to identifying potential airway problems
- Obstructive sleep apnoea is often under diagnosed and can lead to unexpected airway difficulties
- Successful management of the difficult paediatric airway requires meticulous anaesthetic preparation while ensuring minimal distress to the child
- A variety of intubation techniques can be employed using a fibreoptic laryngoscope with and without an exchange catheter.

11.1 Introduction

Major difficulties in managing the paediatric airway arise relatively infrequently and are usually predictable. The incidence of the can't intubate, can't ventilate scenario is fortunately very rare and consequently the anaesthetist who is faced with this eventuality will have had little previous clinical experience of the situation. Anaesthetists have traditionally managed the difficult paediatric airway and intubation using a mixture of basic clinical airway skills and creative techniques, often involving the gum elastic bougie. Until relatively recently the advanced technology for airway manipulation and fibreoptic intubation have been reserved for adult practice. However, the introduction of newer airway devices and high resolution small diameter flexible fibreoptic laryngoscopes, has made the management of children with a difficult airway more controlled and effective.

Unlike adults, the majority of children will not tolerate awake intubation and thus an additional challenge is administration of general anaesthesia and maintaining airway patency while the airway is secured. This chapter describes the anatomy and physiology of the paediatric airway, the recognition of the paediatric difficult airway, both acute and chronic, including syndromic conditions and finally the techniques and equipment that can be used to manage the paediatric difficult airway. Readers who are not experienced in the use of flexible fibreoptic endoscopy and intubation techniques are encouraged to work in tandem with colleagues who regularly undertake these methods in adult practice.

11.2 Differences between adult and paediatric airways – anatomy and physiology

The anatomy of the paediatric airway differs in several fundamental ways from that of the adult. Many of these differences are functionally optimized for sucking and simultaneous swallowing and breathing in the baby and infant. Babies and infants are obligate nose breathers. They have a large head and short neck, which in the supine unconscious infant results in head flexion and airway obstruction. Hyperextension can cause compression of the airway rather than opening it. The tongue in the infant and baby is relatively large and there are often few or no teeth, increasing the risk of airway obstruction within the mouth. The larynx is high at the level of C 3-4 (cf C5–6 in the adult), and the epiglottis is Ω (omega) shaped, relatively large and floppy. In addition, the epiglottis protrudes over the laryngeal inlet at a 45 degree angle. These features favour the use of a straight blade laryngoscope, the tip of which is placed over the epiglottis, up to the age of one year. The narrowest part of the airway is the cricoid ring compared to the laryngeal inlet in adults. Furthermore, the airways are short and narrow so that any reduction in diameter results in a large rise in resistance.

The mechanics of breathing also differ. Babies and preterm babies in particular have horizontal, compressible ribs. The diaphragm, the main respiratory muscle in infancy, consists of a greater proportion of type 2 fibres that fatigue more easily. In addition the abdomen is relatively protuberant and can further impede diaphragmatic function.

Tidal volumes are relatively fixed so that any increase in minute ventilation is achieved by increasing respiratory rate. Oxygen consumption in babies is 6–8 ml/kg/min compared to 3.5 ml/kg/min in the adult. The closing capacity exceeds functional residual capacity (FRC) until at least one year of age. Finally the ratio of alveolar ventilation to FRC is 5:1 in early life, as compared to 1.5:1 in older children and adults. All these factors predispose to rapid hypoxia following interruption in ventilation.

11.3 Recognition of the difficult airway

While there is a lower incidence of the difficult airway in children compared to adults certain clinical conditions and syndromes are known to be associated with airway problems (Table 11.1). Obtaining a good history from the parents is

Table 11.1 Conditions associated with a difficult airway

Syndrome	Specific airway abnormalities
Craniofacial	
Pierre Robin	Cleft Palate, micrognathia, glossoptosios
Treacher Collins	Micrognathia, aplastic zygomatic arches, choanal atresia
Goldenher's	Unilateral facial hypoplasia with mandibular hypoplasia. 40% associated Klippel Feil anomaly
Crouzon's	Craniosynnostosis, hypertelorism, hypoplastic maxilla
Beckwith-Wiedermann	Macroglossia, exophthalamus
Down's syndrome	Macroglossia, small nasopharynx, hypotonia
Lysosomal enzyme defect	
Mucopolysacchoroidoses	A group of disorders (e.g. Hurlers, Scheie's) that lead to progressive thickening of all tissues by partially degraded mucopolysaccharoids
Congenital swellings	
Cystic hygroma	May affect tongue, pharynx and neck
Haemangioma	Can affect tongue as well as lower airway, increases in size until 1–2 years old
Temporomandibular joint/cervical spine problems	
Juvenile Inflammatory Arthritis (Stills disease)	TMJ (ankylosis) and C spine immobility or instability
Cockayne-Touraine	Premature ageing with TMJ ankylosis
Arthrogryposis multiplex	Multiple contractures can lead to reduced mandibular movement
Klippel-Feil	Congenitial fusion of one or more cervical vertebrate making neck movement limited
Acquired pathology	
Tumour	Facial or oropharyngeal
Infection/abscess	Neck, dental, pharyngeal, laryngeal and tracheal
Post radiation	Leads to fibrosis; can cause limited mouth opening
Burns and thermal injury	Initial facial or airway swelling – later contractures

essential in diagnosing a potential difficult airway problem. Parents should be asked whether they have noticed any sleep disturbances and/or excessive snoring suggestive of obstructive sleep apnoea (see below section on OSA), upper airway noises (particularly with reference to position) and whether these increase when the child has an upper respiratory tract infection. Specific enquires should be made about previous anaesthetics and if any problems occurred.

It is not always easy to examine mouth opening and neck movement in children so a certain amount of ingenuity may be required. Careful examination of the child should be performed, both from the front and from the side also noting any dysmorphic features that might be suggestive of a syndrome. In particular look for micrognathia, macroglossia, glossoptosis, small nostrils, facial asymmetry, and any soft tissue mass that might encroach upon the airway. Note any stridor and whether changes in position of the head of the child make it better or worse. Observe the chest, noting any signs of respiratory distress such as recession, retraction and tracheal tug. Examination of the notes, which may be extensive, is at least as important as that of the child; look for any syndrome that may already have been diagnosed and pay particular attention to previous anaesthetic charts which may describe airway problems and how they were overcome. If possible speak to the anaesthetist who cared for the child on the last occasion. Be aware that certain conditions, for example mucopolysaccharoidoses, are progressive so that the degree of airway impairment will worsen with age. Finally, there may have been radiological investigations such as CT scans that can provide useful additional information.

11.4 Obstructive sleep apnoea

Obstructive sleep apnoea (OSA) is increasingly common in children and is frequently under diagnosed. The most common cause of OSA in children is adenotonsillar hypertrophy. Other predisposing factors include craniofacial anomalies, neuromuscular disorders that lead to reduced pharyngeal tone and macroglossia. These features lead to a narrowed upper airway and uncoordinated or decreased pharyngeal tone. This reduced or abnormal pharyngeal muscular activity is unable to counteract the negative intraluminal pressures generated by the respiratory muscles, hence the airway collapses and obstructs.

Identifying OSA in children is not always easy. Typical features include a pattern of night time snoring, followed by silence and then restlessness and awakenings. Daytime somnolence is less commonly seen than in adults; the child is often hyperactive. There may be enuresis, nightmares, morning headaches, and failure to thrive. Longstanding OSA leads to pulmonary hypertension and right ventricular failure. Anaesthetists should always be alert to the possibility of OSA and ask screening questions in the anaesthetic history. If OSA is suspected, initial investigations should include oxygen saturation, an ECG in order to exclude right ventricular hypertrophy and a full blood count to check for polycythaemia. Referal to specialist sleep clinic and further investigations such as echocardiogram, cardiac catheterization and polysomnography may be required.

Definitive management of OSA in children is surgical adenotonsillectomy and an increasing number of children are presenting for this procedure for

Box 11. 1 Features of severe OSA in children

- <2 years of age
- Craniofacial anomalies
- Failure to thrive
- Morbid obesity
- Hypotonia
- Cor pulmonale
- Arterial oxygen desaturation to <70%
- Respiratory disturbance index (number of apnoeas per hour of sleep) >40

relief of OSA symptoms. Children can also present as an emergency, with acute, life threatening obstruction or for incidental surgery with no previous diagnosis of OSA.

Anaesthetic management depends in part on the severity of the OSA. Children with a history of OSA who are at particular risk may have certain features (see Box 11.1).

These children warrant a more cautious approach using the principles described in the relevant section below. Children with OSA, particularly those with severe OSA, are at increased risk of post operative complications. For this reason extubation and recovery should be considered carefully. **Children with severe OSA require a HDU bed or a period of close monitoring in the immediate post operative period**.

11.5 **Stridor and acute airway obstruction**

Acute airway obstruction can be congenital or acquired (see Table 11.2).

Table 11.2 Causes of acute airway obstruction	
Congenital	**Acquired**
Choanal atresia	Laryngotracheobronchitis
Laryngomalacia	Epiglottitis
Laryngeal webs	Tonsillar abscess
Supra/subglottic cysts	Burns
Subglottic stenosis	Post intubation
	Inhaled foreign body

It is important to assess the severity of stridor. Signs of life threatening stridor include decreased consciousness, reduced chest movement (which may lead to little or no stridor), desaturation, periods of apnoea and bradycardia. Clinical concern should lead to a plan to safely secure the airway. Consider using Heliox if it is available – the mixture is of lower density and therefore reduces the work of breathing where airflow is turbulent.

11.6 Anaesthesia

11.6.1 Preoperative preparation (premedication, equipment)

Adequate preparation is the key to successful airway control and intubation in the child with a difficult airway. Obtain the relevant history and gather as much information as possible about the airway from clinical examination, previous notes, and investigations. If the risks of airway management outweigh the necessity for surgery, postponing or cancelling the operation may be appropriate. Discuss the risks with the parents and, if possible, the child, as well as the operating surgeon. If a fibreoptic intubation is planned then specific consent for this should be obtained. It is wise to document all findings and discussion in the notes for future reference – think of the next person who may have to anaesthetize the child.

Consider giving a premedicant. An antimuscarinic can be very useful in both decreasing secretions and the risk of laryngospasm. Traditionally intramuscular atropine 0.02 mg/kg or glycopyrronium bromide 0.005 mg/kg have been used. Alternatively, these drugs can be given orally, in doses of 0.04 mg/kg and 0.10 mg/kg respectively, although in the authors' experience oral administration is less effective. Adequate time is necessary following administration — usually 30–45 minutes, to ensure that production of saliva has ceased and remaining saliva has been swallowed. Anxiolytic sedative medications should generally be avoided.

Ensure a full range of equipment is available – oral and nasal airways, different types (straight and curved) as well as sizes of laryngoscope blades and tracheal tubes plus airway adjuncts such as bougies and stylets. An experienced assistant is essential and a second anaesthetist preferable.

11.6.2 Induction

Most anaesthetists favour the technique of an inhalational induction and maintaining spontaneous ventilation at all times, with the aim of achieving an adequate depth of anaesthesia before performing laryngoscopy and intubation. Sevoflurane or halothane in 100% oxygen are equally effective agents. Position the children so that they are in the most comfortable position at induction, either on a parent's lap or on a trolley. Full monitoring should be applied as soon as it is tolerated by the child. Intravenous access should be obtained either prior to induction with minimal distress to the child or as soon after as possible. Obstruction of the airway may occur as soon as the child loses consciousness but prior to a depth of anaesthesia that permits laryngoscopy. Various strategies can be used to overcome the obstruction. Maintaining continuous positive airway pressure (CPAP) via a close fitting face mask and partially occluded bag of an Ayre's-T- piece is often helpful. Turning the child to the lateral or even prone position can also be valuable. Care should be taken in using an orophyngeal airway in too light a plane of anaesthesia; a nasophyngeal airway may be better tolerated at this stage. If the child does become apnoeic or begins to cough, resist the temptation to assist ventilation. Oxygenation can usually be maintained with CPAP while waiting for spontaneous ventilation to resume. Insertion of a laryngeal mask airway (LMA) can also be useful in opening the airway and delivering sufficient volatile to deepen the patient. If it proves impossible to adequately maintain the airway then it is no disgrace to wake the child up and reconsider the options available. If this is not an option either cricothyroidotomy or surgical tracheostomy should be considered.

11.7 Methods of intubation

11.7.1 Conventional

This method for intubation using a rigid laryngoscope is generally used for children with glottic or subglottic partial airway obstruction such as epiglottis and laryngotracheobronchitis.

When a sufficient depth of anaesthesia has been reached, position the child carefully for laryngoscopy. Neonates and infants may benefit from a roll under the shoulders and need a neutral head position. Older children may need a pillow and more neck flexion. If prolonged attempts at intubation are anticipated oxygen can be given via a nasal prong or via an adapted laryngoscope.

In addition to conventional laryngoscopes such as the straight Robertshaw or curved Mackintosh, modified paediatric size laryngoscopes are available such as the McCoy. Cricoid pressure is an invaluable manoeuvre which when directed posteriorly and to the right often provides the best views. Gum elastic bougies or stylets can help negotiate an awkward oropharynx angle. A large tongue can be retracted using McGill forceps by an assistant. Insertion of dental roll into a cleft palate can also aid laryngoscopy. Be aware that prolonged attempts at intubation will result in the child lightening from anaesthesia. Thus it is important to return to facemask anaesthesia at frequent intervals. Again, if it proves impossible to intubate, then waking the child up should be considered.

11.7.2 Fibreoptic laryngoscope intubation

Fibreoptic intubation has now become an accepted technique in children and is frequently the preferred method in the anticipated paediatric difficult airway particularly in children with supraglottic airway obstruction.

There are several sizes of fibreoptic laryngoscope available. The smallest has an external diameter of 2.0 mm and will allow the passage of a 2.5 mm tracheal tube (TT). It has no side channel for suction or for giving local anaesthetic. In addition it is quite flexible which makes it difficult to manipulate. The next size up, which does have a side channel, has a diameter of 2.8 mm; it is stiffer and easier to use and will allow passage of a 3.0 mm TT. Fibreoptic intubation can be performed via the nasal or oral routes. The nasal route rarely causes bleeding in children and provides a good angle of approach and view of the larynx. The oral route can be harder to negotiate and may require adapted oropharyngeal airways or LMA to provide access to the larynx (Figure 11.1).

Children with reduced movement at the temporomandibular joint or very poor mouth opening will invariably require a nasal intubation.

11.7.3 Fibreoptic intubation via conventional airway methods

Oxygenation and anaesthesia can be maintained either with a nasal prong/ airway, or an adapted face mask (Figure 11.2). It is preferable to have two anaesthetists, one to manage the airway and ventilation and the other to perform the fibreoptic intubation.

It is usually unnecessary to tropicalize the nose in younger children if a nasal intubation is planned. However, it can be valuable to apply local anaesthetic to the larynx and trachea prior to intubation to prevent coughing and laryngospasm. The fibreoptic laryngoscope can be inserted either via the nose or via an adapted oropharyngeal airway and facemask. (Figure 11.3), (Figure 11.4). Once the larynx and trachea have been visualized, an epidural catheter can be inserted via the side port and lidocaine 3 mg/kg can be dropped on to the larynx and between the cords.

Two basic techniques for fibreoptic intubation can then be employed. The simplest is the 'TT over fibreoptic scope technique' where an appropriately sized TT is preloaded onto the fibreoptic scope and the TT is passed into the

Figure 11.1 Modified paediatric oropharyngeal airways that can be used for fibreoptic intubation

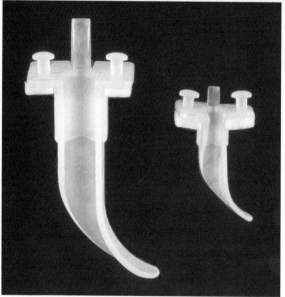

Reproduced with permission of Oxford Medical Illustration (OMI).

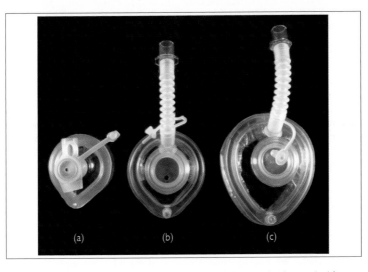

Figure 11.2 Adapted right angle connector with silicone seal cap used with a standard face mask [a] and two sizes of adapted face masks [b, c] which permit insertion of a fibreoptic laryngoscope.

Reproduced with permission of Oxford Medical Illustration (OMI).

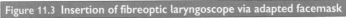

Figure 11.3 Insertion of fibreoptic laryngoscope via adapted facemask

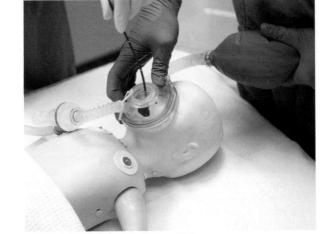

Reproduced with permission of Oxford Medical Illustration (OMI).

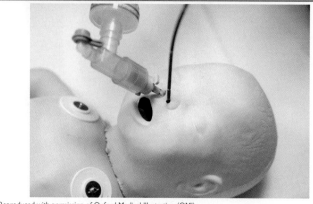

Figure 11.4 Nasal airway to maintain anaesthesia in opposite nostril to insertion of fibrescope

Reproduced with permission of Oxford Medical Illustration (OMI).

trachea under direct visualization. However, if the TT is the wrong size, the procedure has to be repeated, risking increased trauma to the airway. The second technique is a 'guidewire/exchange catheter technique' where a flexible tipped guidewire is passed into the trachea, via the fibreoptic scope side channel (not possible with the 2.0 mm scope). Once the guidewire is in the trachea, the fibreoptic scope can be removed. An exchange catheter can be passed over the wire to stiffen it and a TT then railroaded over the catheter (Figure 11.5). A variation of the technique is to load the exchange catheter itself onto the scope – a 2.0 mm scope will accept an 11 mm exchange catheter. The exchange catheter technique has several advantages. The exchange catheter can be used to oxygenate/ventilate the patient, as well as to verify position using capnography. It allows the trial of different size TT with minimal trauma and prevents the need for repeated passing of the fibreoptic scope. If the fibrescope being used is too large to pass into the trachea, the fibrescope can be positioned just above the larynx and then the guidewire placed into the trachea. This is a safe and flexible method for intubation.

11.7.4 Fibreoptic intubation through an LMA

The LMA is becoming an essential tool in the management of a difficult airway in modern paediatric anaesthetic practice. It can be used to manage an airway when the child is obstructing but not yet deep enough for laryngoscopy, as discussed above. It can also be used as a conduit for fibreoptic intubation (if an oral TT is acceptable) while maintaining anaesthesia via the LMA. Following insertion of the LMA adequate time is required to deepen anaesthesia to permit intubation and establish spontaneous respiration. A specially adapted right angle connector with silicone seal cap can be used to connect to the LMA to permit insertion of the

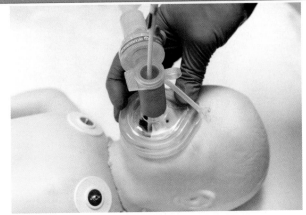

Figure 11.5 Rail roading TT over exchange catheter through adapted right angle connector

Reproduced with permission of Oxford Medical Illustration (OMI).

fibreoptic scope and allow an airtight seal. The fibreoptic scope can be passed down the LMA and the cords visualised. Local anaesthetic can be applied as previously described. The two methods for fibreoptic intubation can then be used as previously described:

1. The TT over fibreoptic scope technique (Figure 11.6). Care must be taken in removing the LMA once the child has been intubated. A half size smaller TT can be inserted into the proximal end of the intubation TT and gentle pressure applied as the LMA is removed (Figure 11.7).

2. The guidewire/exchange catheter technique. This is the only method that can be used with an armoured TT where it is not possible to remove the 11 mm connector. (Figure 11.8). In these circumstances the LMA can be removed before intubation, after the exchange catheter has been inserted. The advantage of guidewire technique when using an LMA is that the guidewire can be left in place until the LMA is removed and position of the TT is confirmed, in case of accidental extubation.

If surgical access to the mouth is not required and the TT is long enough the LMA can be left in place.

For peace of mind, whichever fibreoptic intubation technique is used, it is always helpful to finally confirm the position of the TT in the trachea using the fibrescope.

11.8 Can't intubate, can't ventilate

As mentioned above, there are no figures for the incidence of this scenario within the paediatric population but it is fortunately rare. Maintaining

Figure 11.6 Insertion of fibrescope through LMA with TT attached

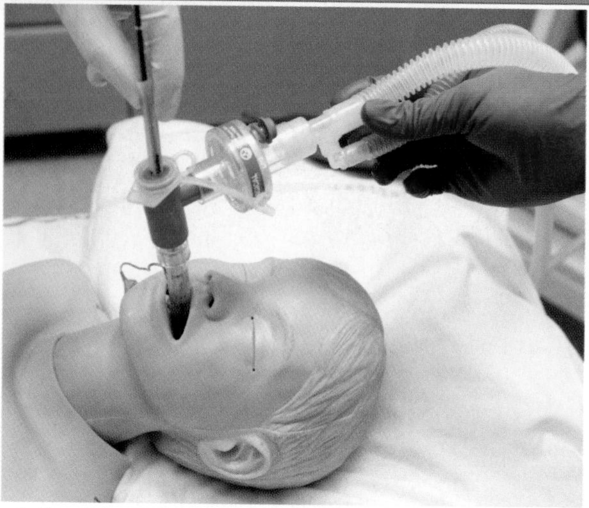

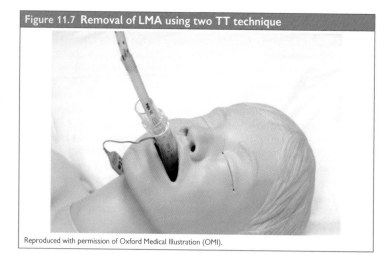

Reproduced with permission of Oxford Medical Illustration (OMI).

Figure 11.7 Removal of LMA using two TT technique

Reproduced with permission of Oxford Medical Illustration (OMI).

Figure 11.8 Insertion of exchange catheter over guidewire through LMA

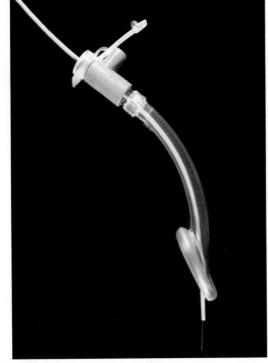

Reproduced with permission of Oxford Medical Illustration (OMI).

oxygenation is of paramount importance and if there is no alternative, needle cricothyroidotomy is the last resort. Having experienced help is invaluable if faced with this situation.

The paediatric trachea is narrow (5 mm diameter in the infant), the larynx higher and the cricothyroid membrane more difficult to palpate. A 16 or 14G cannula, or specifically designed cricothyriodotomy catheter set using a Seldinger guidewire technique can be used in infants and prepubertal children. These can be connected to an oxygen source via a Luer lock or 15 mm connector. Ventilating through these devices requires a higher flow of oxygen than a self inflating bag can provide. The oxygen source can be attached via a 3 way tap or Y piece connector. Start the flow at the age of the child in years in L/min. Occlude the Y piece or 3 way tap for 1 second and observe for rise of the chest; if there is insufficient movement, cautiously increase the flow. Alternatively, if there is a pressurised source of oxygen, limit initial inflation to 1kPa. Expiration cannot occur through the cannula or catheter. Therefore the child must exhale through the upper airway even if it is partially obstructed. Allow enough time for expiration and be aware of the dangers of air trapping, rising pressures, and resultant barotrauma.

11.9 **Extubation and recovery**

Extubation is as important to consider and plan for as intubation. In general, the child with the difficult airway should be fully awake before extubation. Some anaesthetists prefer to extubate asleep and spontaneously breathing. It is argued that this leads to better recovery conditions with less coughing and risk of bleeding. An oral or nasopharyngeal airway can be helpful in this scenario. However, the reduced pharyngeal tone may cause airway obstruction.

If planning an awake extubation the child should be completely reversed from the muscle relaxant. One well-known mantra is to wait until you think the child is ready for extubation, then wait for another 20 breaths. The child should be placed in the position that is most comfortable for the child but is also easiest for the anaesthetist to support the airway. All equipment and drugs used for the initial intubation should be readily available. If airway surgery has been performed, the airway should be visually inspected prior to extubation.

Recovery should be in an area with emergency paediatric intubation equipment available. Experienced staff should be available who are able to identify and initially manage the airway in a child who is struggling. Those children at higher risk, for example the child with severe OSA, should be monitored in a high dependency area for 24 hours. Close observations need to be made for signs of oversedation, opiate induced hypoventilation, and apnoeas.

11.10 **New ventilation and intubation devices**

In the last five years there has been a plethora of novel supraglottic airway devices and equipment to visualize the airway. Most of these have only been developed for adult use. However, it is likely that in the near future some of these will be produced in paediatric sizes. One of most promising supraglottic airway devices in the view of the authors is the i-gel (Intersurgical, Wickingham, Berkshire RG41 2RZ, UK). This has a soft gel-like non inflatable cuff which conforms to the shape of the perilaryngeal anatomy forming a seal. The cuff is connected to a tube that incorporates a bite block which passes through the oropharynx and mouth. It appears to be relatively easy to insert and could be used as an alternative to the LMA for airway maintenance and as a conduit to fibreoptic intubation. Other aids to intubation include the Bullard laryngoscope which is a ridge laryngoscope that is inserted blindly and using fibreoptics allows a view of the larynx. A TT can be passed via a ridge stylet. A paediatric size is available and has proved useful. Various other ridged laryngoscopes based on the principle of the Bullard have been also developed including the Glidescope (Verathon Medical, Aylesbury, Buckinghamshire, HP17

8JB, UK) and Airtraq (Frannin Ltd, Reading, Berkshire, RG31 7SB, UK). These are disposable devices and use conventional mirrors and optics to view the laryngeal inlet. Paediatric sizes are now available.

Appendix

Examples of equipment suitable for paediatric difficult intubation:

Appendix	
Equipment	**Manufacturer**
Paediatric fibre-optic laryngoscope 2.0 mm and 2.8 mm	Karl Storz Endoscopy Ltd
Infant child adapted paediatric facemasks (VBM endoscopy masks)	Freelance Surgical Ltd
Infant and child adapted (split) oropharyngeal airways VBM	Freelance Surgical Ltd
11 mm rught angle connector with rubber seal to connect to facemask/LMA TT Mianz (Roush) Adaptors	Karl Storz Endoscopy Ltd
Airway Excvhange Catheters: Paediatric 8.0–45 × 4 Paediatric 11.0–8.3 × 4	Cook Medical Ltd
Intubating Introducers Paediatric 8.3–35 × 2 Frova	Cook Medical Ltd
Guidewires Straight tip TSF .38–145–0.038 in J TIP TSF –38–145–3 0.038 in	Cook Medical Ltd
Cricothyroidotomy set Meiker Emergency Cricothyroidotomy Catheter Sete 3.5 & 4 mm	Cook Medical Care Ltd

Further reading

Brouillette R, Hanson D, David R. A diagnostic approach to suspected obstructive sleep apnoea in children. *Journal of paediatrics* 1984; **105**: 10–14.

Cardwell M, Walker RWM. Management of the difficult paediatric airway. *BJA/CEPD reviews* 2003; **3**(6):167–70.

Frank Y, Kravath RE, Pollak CP, Weitzman ED. Obstructive sleep apnoea and its therapy: clinical and polysomnographic manifestations. *Paediatrics* 1983; **71**: 737–42.

Thomas PB, Parry MG. The difficult paediatric airway: a new method of fibreoptic intubation using the laryngeal mask, Cook airway exchange catheter and tracheal induction fibrescope. *Paediatric Anaesthesia* 2001; **11**: 618–21.

Walker RWM. The laryngeal mask airway in the difficult airway: an assessment of positioning and use in fibreoptic intubation. *Paediatric Anaesthesia* 2000; **10**: 53–8.

Warwick JP, Mason DG. Obstructive sleep apnoea syndrome in children. *Anaesthesia* 1998; **53**: 571–9.

Chapter 12

Extubation and re-intubation strategy

Ravi Dravid and Gene Lee

Key points

- Airway complications occur more frequently at and following extubation than at intubation
- Complications at extubation can have catastrophic consequences
- Conditions for airway management at extubation are less than ideal
- Extubation is an elective procedure and should be controlled
- It is possible to risk stratify extubation and plan a safe strategy
- Appropriate techniques for the 'High risk' extubation allow oxygenation and safe re intubation.

12.1 Introduction

Limited UK data suggests that the incidence of airway complications at extubation is as high as 12.6% and is 2.5 times more than that occurring at induction of anaesthesia. US data suggests that closed claims arising from morbidity and mortality during induction of anaesthesia has recently seen a significant reduction but has remained the same at extubation. The incidence of failed extubation requiring re-intubation after routine anaesthesia is 0.2% and as high as 20% in the ITU setting. It is especially high after pan-endoscopy, head and neck surgery and possibly in the obese and those with obstructive sleep apnoea (OSA). Failed extubation in ITU accounts for a high in-hospital mortality.

This chapter introduces the concept of 'decision-outcome analysis'—a method for planning and risk stratifying extubation into low, intermediate or high risk. Techniques of extubation for each risk category are discussed with particular emphasis on the use of devices that can be used for oxygenation and re intubation of 'high risk' patients.

12.2 Complications at extubation

12.2.1 Mostly minor
- breath holding and transient laryngospasm;
- coughing;
- teeth clenching/masseter spasm;
- dental/oral/pharyngeal damage;
- laryngeal injury;
- paradoxical vocal cord movement (PVCM).

12.2.2 Major
- severe laryngospasm leading to hypoxia or negative pressure pulmonary oedema (NPPO);
- airway obstruction, loss of airway, hypoxia and brain injury;
- regurgitation, aspiration or airway soiling;
- Hypertensive responses and cardiovascular instability.

12.3 Why is extubation hazardous?

12.3.1 Anaesthesia adversely affects airway patency, ventilation and gas exchange
- Impaired airway patency:
  - active airway obstruction due to laryngospasm or cord dysfunction;
  - passive airway obstruction from reduced pharyngeal tone or pharyngeal collapse as in the obese or in those with OSA.
- Airway reactivity:
  - Normal airway reflexes become excessive or difficult to manage in lighter planes of anaesthesia leading to coughing, breath-holding or laryngospasm.
- Impaired oxygen stores: limited oxygen stores are very rapidly depleted.
  - Pre-oxygenation at extubation is less efficient when compared to induction.
  - The wash-in of high FiO2 is impaired by:
  - Altered pulmonary function.
  - Diffusion hypoxia.
  - Breaking the circuit when moving the patient replaces high FiO2 with air.
  - Time period of pre-oxygenation 'limited' by emergence.
- Rapid depletion of oxygen stores and rapid de-saturation as in children and the obese.

12.3.2 Unfavourable conditions at extubation reduce access to the airway and reduce the time available to intervene and prevent or reverse hypoxia

- Practical difficulties with establishing ventilation.
- Mask ventilation is likely to be challenging especially in an agitated, hypoxic patient recovering from the anaesthetic. Conditions for re-intubation are likely to be worse than at induction especially if it has been difficult or traumatic.
- Altered anatomy: (Either physical or mechanical limitation to airway access or actual pathological distortion of airway due to injury, surgery or disease).
  - Bony or soft tissue impediments (preoperative abnormality of face, mouth, jaw or cervical spine or surgical fixation, implants, etc.).
  - Airway access – shared airway/wiring or surgical fixation/guardian sutures.
  - Pre-existing airway abnormality – tumour/swelling/congenital/scarring-surgery/burns/radiotherapy.
  - Post airway surgery or trauma – airway oedema/tracheomalacia/swelling/bleeding or haematoma/nerve injury and laryngeal injuries. Note: neck haematoma causes supra and peri-glottic oedema due to lymphatic and venous obstruction, which makes intubation difficult even after its drainage.

12.3.3 Aspiration and airway soiling

- Incidence of aspiration at extubation is difficult to quantify.
- The risk is increased with CNS surgery, bulbar, cranial nerve palsies.
- Debris, surgical gauze and instruments pose foreign body risk.
- Upper airway bleeding will pool with gravity and later aspirated, aided by inspiratory efforts of the patient.

12.3.4 Other factors

- Impaired respiratory drive and ventilation from residual drug effects and inadequate neuromuscular function.
- Mechanical restrictions from thoracic or abdominal splinting.
- Impaired cardiovascular, neurological function, temperature, fluid, electrolyte, and acid base status.

12.3.5 Equipment failure and human factors

- These factors can result from distraction, time pressures, and operator fatigue.

> Managing extubation:
> **Important!! Extubation is an elective episode. Plan it well.**
> Successful airway management at extubation requires a 'Decision-Outcome analysis'. This has following steps:

Decision – outcome analysis

Step 1 – Survey

    a)   Pre-Extubation Review (PER)

    b)   Ease of airway access at extubation

To determine the ease or success at extubation

This allows…

Step 2 – Risk stratification

Into low, intermediate and high risk extubation

This helps to devise an appropriate…

Step 3 – Extubation strategy

Customized for low / intermediate / high risk extubation

12.4 **Decision-outcome analysis**

Step 1 Survey – before each extubation perform:

    a). Pre-Extubation Review (PER)

    b). Evaluate ease of airway access at extubation

A: Pre-Extubation Review (PER):
Assess the following to minimize the risk of extubation failure

- Adequate airway patency, stable pulmonary function, spontaneous and normal respiratory pattern.
- Adequate or normally progressing neurological and neuro-muscular recovery.
- A stable cardio-vascular, metabolic, electrolyte, temperature status.
- Absent abdominal or thoracic splinting effect.
- The level of recovery for each of these factors does not necessarily advance in tandem and must be individually assessed.

B: Evaluate ease of airway access at extubation:
ASK

> **Was the airway normal/uncomplicated at induction and does it continue to be the same?**

Scenarios:

- **No change**:

Was normal at induction and remains normal/easy by the end of surgery.

- **Operative restrictions:**

Was normal at induction but access to airway limited by the end of surgery- shared airway, head or neck fixation, e.g. halos, wires, surgical implants, cervical spine fixation.

- **Intra-operative worsening:**
Was normal at induction but may have become difficult e.g. altered/distorted anatomy from bleeding, haematoma, and swelling, oedema due to surgery, trauma or non-surgical factors.

- **Pre-existing difficulties:**
Known difficult airway at induction – either previously anticipated or unanticipated at induction. Includes obesity and obstructive sleep apnoea. The airway may or may not have worsened intraoperatively.

Step 2 – Risk stratification

The **survey (step 1)** allows classification into low / intermediate / high risk

PER	INITIAL AIRWAY	EASE OF AIRWAY ACCESS	RISK
Satisfactory	Normal	Assured	Low
Doubtful	Normal	Assured	Intermediate
Satisfactory	Normal	Doubtful	High
Satisfactory	Difficult	Doubtful	High

Note: Extubation may fail for a number of medical, surgical and anaesthetic reasons. The proposed risk stratification is based on the ability to rapidly re-establish a patent airway and effective ventilation and oxygenation.

Step 3 – Extubation strategy

There is no evidence presently to support the use of an extubation strategy; however there is an overwhelming consultant opinion which favours that a pre-formulated 'extubation strategy' should be in place. Step 2 allows this to be planned as follows:

RISK	EXTUBATION STRATEGY
Low	– Routine extubation
	– Provide continuous oxygen through routine low flow devices
Intermediate	– Trial extubation, re-intubation achievable rapidly
	– Routine extubation with continuous high flow/100% oxygen
High	– Re-intubation may be difficult or not achievable rapidly
	– Use a technique that allows a continuous supply of oxygen and rapid re-intubation should extubation fail.

12.5 **Extubation strategy**

12.5.1 **General principles**

- Plan extubation in a suitable location with at least the same level of airway equipment, monitoring, and skilled help as at initial intubation.
- Build adequate oxygen stores before extubation.
- Ensure minimum interruption in supply of oxygen at all stages.
- Integrate a rescue plan for rapid re-intubation should extubation fail.

12.5.2 **Pre-oxygenation**

- Pre-oxygenation at induction requires a 3–5 minute 100% oxygenation period during spontaneous ventilation. At emergence, variable tidal volumes and impaired pulmonary function due to anaesthesia may hinder the normal wash-in of oxygenation. There is no evidence to suggest the ideal duration, but the aim is to achieve FeO_2 as close to FiO_2 as possible similar to the pre-induction phase.
- Initial controlled ventilation with 100% oxygen may speed this process.

12.5.3 **Position-Supine vs. lateral head down vs. head-up**

- Evidence is lacking to support a universal extubation position.
- A left lateral head down position has been termed as 'evidence based' for extubating the non-fasted patient.
- There is increasing trend towards undertaking extubation in a fasted patient in a supine position or supine with a slight head up tilt especially in obese population. This allows mechanical advantage for respiration and perhaps also better re-intubating conditions.

12.5.4 **Depth-Awake versus deep extubation**

- Extubation should be carried out at the appropriate depth or recovery of airway reflexes suitable for patient and surgical requirements.
- Traditional wisdom has been to extubate either fully 'awake' or 'deep'.
- Awake extubation is generally safer as the return of airway tone, reflexes and respiratory drive allows the patient to manage and maintain their own airway.
- There is mixed evidence for the use of deep extubation. Deep extubation may avoid adverse cardiovascular and respiratory responses especially in surgical procedures where coughing and straining is undesirable. This needs to be balanced with an overall increase in the incidence of early and late airway complications.

12.5.5 **Low risk extubation strategy or routine extubation**

- PER normal, initial airway normal and patency at extubation assured if re-intubation is required.
- Standard awake or deep technique with low flow oxygen supplementation for recovery.

12.5.6 **Technique of awake extubation**

- Appropriated pre-oxygenation / pre-extubation oxygenation.
- Supply oxygen through the breathing system continuously.
- Suction oropharynx under direct vision – suctioning blindly can result in airway trauma.
- Allow emergence and establishment of regular pattern of breathing.
- Deflate tracheal tube cuff and assess response – response to cuff deflation can be a re-assuring sign of an adequate return of airway reflexes but may also be an indication of secretions or debris above the tube and thus the need for further suctioning.
- Minimize head and neck movements.
- Apply positive pressure and extubate – this helps recruitment of alveoli, expels pooled secretions and reduces likelihood of post-extubation laryngeal spasm which has traditionally been reported to occur in the expiratory phase of breathing.
- Follow with oxygen supplementation – various low or high flow devices or CPAP.
- Adjuvant drugs: lidocaine-spray or intravenous, beta-blockers, propofol, glyceryl trinitrate, titrated dose of opioids are options to facilitate tube tolerance.

12.5.7 **Suggested deep extubation technique**

- Removal of tracheal tube before recovery of laryngeal reflexes.
- Ensure that there is no further surgical stimulation.
- Balance of adequate analgesia while not overtly inhibiting respiratory drive.
- Alveolar should be maximized by removing nitrous oxide and an adequate anaesthetic depth maintained by increasing inspired concentration of inhalational agent.
- Position patient in left lateral or supine with minimal movement of head or tracheal tube.
- Suction and deflate cuff and demonstrate no airway response such as cough, gag or a change in breathing pattern. Responses may indicate an intermediate depth of anaesthesia and a need to deepen the anaesthetic plane.
- Positive pressure while still administering inhalational agent and extubate.
- Keep airway patent with either an oral or naso-pharyngeal airway.
- Oxygen supplementation and close monitoring till full recovery of consciousness.
- Adjuncts/Additional techniques – supra-glottic airway devices such as a laryngeal mask airway can be supplemented for recovery and 'mask free' ventilation if required in special surgical situations.

12.5.8 **Intermediate risk extubation strategy**

- Where PER casts a doubt on the possible success of extubation. In this case a trial extubation is being attempted in a patient with a normal airway.
- Readiness of rapid re-intubation (consider location, equipment, skilled manpower, and monitoring)
- Any of above techniques may be used.
- Oxygen supplementation devices – ensure continuous supply of oxygen with high flow/CPAP.
- Continue to manage post-anaesthetic care in an appropriate area while a need for possible re-intubation exists.

12.5.9 **High-risk extubation strategy**

- Pre extubation review should be optimized.
- Initial airway normal or difficult.
- Ease of airway access at extubation doubtful.

12.6 **Techniques for high-risk extubation**

a). Awake extubation with a rescue plan worked out in advance.

b). Extubation with rescue devices.

A rescue device is inserted *before* removal of tracheal tube. Recovery takes place with the device in place allowing continuous oxygenation and rapid re-intubation if required. Rescue devices are mostly tolerated without additional sedation or local anaesthesia. Numerous techniques based on risk/benefit and operator familiarity have been described in the literature. Some are discussed below.

12.6.1 **Supra-glottic airway devices (SADs)**

The tracheal tube is substituted with an appropriate supra glottic device before extubation. The advantages are:

- Maintains a patent airway, allows ventilation if necessary and permits gradual emergence and establishment of own airway.
- Potential for less airway irritation, coughing, and cardiovascular stress response.
- Potentially smoother recovery profile.
- Provides a conduit for fibre optic assessment of airway patency and cord function.
- May be used as a dedicated airway for re-intubation.

12.6.1.1 *Indications*

- Obese and patients with OSA.
- Conduit for evaluation of vocal cord function and route guide for re-intubation/exchange catheter insertion.
- Skin graft to neck and face: avoid mask ventilation and compression of vessels.

- Head and neck surgery: avoid hypertension, bleeding, airway obstruction.
- Open eye surgery: avoid face mask ventilation, severe coughing.
- ENT surgery: prevents airway soiling and obstruction.

12.6.1.2 *Disadvantages*

- May delay awakening.
    - — Laryngospasm during recovery from anaesthesia.
    - — Malposition of LMA may cause airway obstruction.

12.6.1.3 *SAD substitution technique*

For slides of technique please visit www.orag.co.uk/book.

- Clear airway of secretions.
- Insert the supra-glottic device (LMA/ProSeal) behind the tracheal tube. This will minimize the risk of losing the airway in between substituting devices.
- Confirm optimum placement, inspect patency with fibreoptic scope.
- Reverse neuromuscular block, establish spontaneous respiration and remove tracheal tube under direct vision.
- Continue spontaneous respiration with 100% oxygen through LMA to full recovery.
- Re-intubation can be achieved by deepening plane of anaesthesia and utilizing fibreoptic scope to pass tracheal tube or exchange catheter through the SAD (LMA).

12.6.2 Infra-glottic devices

> **Devices placed in the trachea before removal of the tracheal tube to facilitate rapid oxygenation and re-intubation if extubation fails**

Several devices have been used and include: naso-gastric tube, gum-elastic bougie, obturator, introducer, tube exchangers, endo-tracheal ventilation catheter (ETVC).
An ideal device should:

- allow continuous oxygen insufflation or jet ventilation to prevent hypoxia when extubation fails or during re-intubation;
- allow spontaneous ventilation around it;
- permit CO_2 monitoring;
- be left in situ for many hours post-extubation until threat of extubation failure exists;
- facilitate re-intubation by allowing a tracheal tube to be railroaded.

Devices that can be used as Endo Tracheal Ventilation Catheter – available in the UK:

- Aintree Intubation Catheter* (see Chapter 7):
    - 19F with 4.8 mm inner diameter;
    - allows rail-roading of tubes 7.0 mm and greater;
    - allows passage of fibreoptic scope through the inner lumen.

---

* These catheters also have Rapi Fit adaptors for connection to a jet ventilator.

- FROVA bougie:
  - 14F with inner lumen, rounded tip and side ports;
  - permits rail-roading of tracheal tubes 5.0 mm and greater
- Cook Paediatric Airway Exchange catheters*:
  - available in 8F (allows 3 mm tube), 11F (allows 4.0 mm tube), 14F (allows 5.0 mm tube).
- Cook Extra Firm Airway catheter*:
  - 11F and 14F. Made of plastic therefore less compliant.

12.6.3 **Airway Exchange Catheter Technique**

12.6.3.1 *Catheter design and placement*

- Side ports decrease distal lumen pressure and whip with jet ventilation.
- Narrow bore devices are generally better tolerated; those with a larger bore are better for railroading.
- Locate its tip via tracheal tube in the mid trachea and away from the carina, avoiding the main bronchus; this improves catheter tolerance and safety during jet ventilation.
- Tracheal tube is removed over the catheter.
- Securely tape the catheter at the angle of the mouth to prevent its distal migration.
- Leave it in situ until the need for possible re-intubation has passed.
- Supply/insufflate oxygen with a low-pressure system.
- Still permits simultaneous phonation and nebulisation or Heliox administration if required.
- Reasonable patient tolerance has been demonstrated despite apparent stiffness of devices.
- Tolerance can be improved by minimum head movement, opioids, lidocaine, or small doses of propofol.

12.6.3.2 *Managing jet ventilation via exchange catheters*

- Primary aim should be to prevent or reverse life threatening hypoxia rather than full ventilation.
- High pressure jet ventilation with an in-line pressure reducing system, e.g. ManuJet III™ allow pressure settings from the neonatal to the adult range.
- Begin at the lowest setting that will produce chest expansion. It is recommended to start at 1 bar for adults and work slowly upwards.
- Unobstructed expiration is essential for safe jet ventilation.
- Perform basic airway manoeuvres such as jaw thrust, neck extension and ensure an unobstructed upper airway with airway aids if required.
- Allow adequate expiratory time to permit the egress of expired gas to full chest deflation. Failure to allow for unimpeded expiration risks breath stacking and barotrauma.

12.6.4 Cricothyroidotomy/transtracheal surgical devices

- Cannula cricothyroidectomy – A narrow bore cricothyroid cannula (e.g. Ravussin) is placed and its position verified before tracheal tube is removed. If extubation fails then jet ventilation is performed through the cannula until a definitive airway is restored.
- Surgical airway – consider tracheostomy under surgical conditions before awakening.

12.6.5 Delay extubation

- If reversible factors present or recovery conditions not optimal consider elective sedation and ventilation in a critical care setting.
- 8 mg IV dexamethasone 8hrly should prove useful.
- Reassess with cuff deflated for adequate leak around tracheal tube.
- Fibre optic evaluation may help before extubation.

12.7 Problems of special significance at extubation

12.7.1 Laryngospasm

- Transient or sustained bilateral adduction of vocal cords outlasting stimulus and may be associated with masseter spasm.
- Recognized triggers include laryngeal or vocal cord stimulation or non-airway triggers such as vagal, trigeminal, splanchnic, and phrenic nerve stimulation.
- Greatest risk if extubation is attempted in the expiration phase or in a plane between deep and awake.
- Variable severity from stridor to complete airway obstruction; if unrelieved can result in hypoxia, negative pressure pulmonary oedema (NPPO), brain damage or death.

12.7.2 Management of post extubation laryngeal spasm

12.7.2.1 *Prevention*

- Avoid airway or non-airway triggers.
- Visual airway inspection if in doubt or in special situations.
- Choose appropriate depth for extubation – deep or awake.
- Avoid excessive head or neck movements.
- Remove tracheal tube in the inspiratory phase or with a squeeze of reservoir bag.

12.7.2.2 *Recognition*

- Stridor.
- Marked supra-sternal withdrawing.
- Masseter spasm.

- Minimal or no movement of air despite inspiratory efforts or positive pressure ventilation.
- Rapid desaturation.
- Regurgitation of gastric contents could both be cause or result of laryngospasm.

12.7.2.3 *Treatment*

- Alert extra and skilled help.
- Consider other causes of severe airway obstruction.
- Remove airway and non-airway triggers.
- Deliver facemask ventilation with 100% oxygen and CPAP; if spasm persists attempt two-operator mask ventilation.
- If no response, attempt Larson's manoeuvre-jaw thrust with point stimulation behind TMJ. Two fingers are placed on each side of the jaw, in front of the tragus of the ear on the posterior border of the ramus of the mandible. The jaw is pulled forward and downwards.
- If the spasm is unrelieved and oxygen saturation continues to fall, possible courses of action include:
  1. Deepen the anaesthetic with intravenous propofol. This drug relaxes the muscular tissues of the upper respiratory tract and allows ventilation of the lungs with 100% oxygen. An appropriate dose is unknown at present; a large dose is potentially cardiac depressant and could be catastrophic in a hypoxic patient.
  2. Suxamethonium Chloride – A 0.1 mg.kg^{-1} dose intravenously produces partial paralysis and adequate relaxation of vocal cords to permit ventilation.
  3. Tracheal re-intubation.
  4. Trans-tracheal access – cricothyroidotomy.

12.7.3 **Post extubation cord dysfunction**

- May be asymptomatic or present with:
  - impaired phonation – hoarse voice;
  - poor cough;
  - dysphagia, aspiration or subclinical aspiration;
  - stridor or respiratory difficulties.
- A variety of possible causes:
  - paradoxical vocal cord motion;
  - recurrent laryngeal nerve injury;
  - traumatic injury to the cords.
- Paradoxical vocal cord motion (PVCM):
  - mechanism not well understood;
  - direct laryngoscopy reveals vocal cord adduction on inspiration which results in inspiratory stridor; may necessitate re-intubation;
  - appears to be a functional abnormality which may be associated with anxiety during the recovery from anaesthesia;

- calming and re-assuring patients, the use of sedation with propofol or a slow emergence with a gradual reduction with TIVA infusions has been used.
- Assessment:
  - fibre optic nasendoscopy-Fibre optic examination via the nose is well tolerated. Asymmetrical or adducted cords seen;
  - direct laryngoscopy/microlaryngoscopy under anaesthesia-cricoarytenoid joints looking for disarticulation;
  - ENT review.
- Treatment:
  - minor cases can be observed in HDU setting;
  - moderate cases can be managed with facemask CPAP to stent cords open if recovery is possible;
  - re-intubation if severe.

12.7.4 Aspiration/regurgitation on extubation

12.7.4.1 *Immediate at regurgitation*

- Head down tilt to limit pulmonary aspiration and apply pharyngeal suction to remove obvious particulate matter.
- Further response dependent on severity and level of recovery.
- Regurgitation in light plane could result in laryngospasm and thus limit amount aspirated into the trachea.
- It could also result from sustained negative intra-thoracic pressure due to inspiratory effort against a closed glottis.

12.7.4.2 *If minor aspiration*

- Apply facemask oxygen and recover in head down position.
- Assess for laryngospasm, bronchospasm, cyanosis, pulmonary oedema and treat appropriately.
- Development of respiratory failure may require re-intubation.
- Patients may be discharged to general ward if asymptomatic 2 hours post aspiration.

12.7.4.3 *If major aspiration or deep plane of anaesthesia and risk of further aspiration*

- Apply cricoid pressure.
- Re-intubation to prevent further aspiration.
- Consider NG tube if airway secured to empty stomach.
- Bronchospasm, chemical pneumonitis, pulmonary oedema, and CVS collapse may develop and treated with usual supportive therapy.
- Delayed complications include aspiration pneumonia.
- There is no evidence supporting empirical antibiotics or routine steroid treatment. Differentiate from pneumonitis and pneumonia to treat infection in a targeted way.
- Bronchoscopy to assess soiling, apply bronchial lavage and remove particulate material.

Further reading

Arndt GA, Voth BR: Paradoxical vocal cord motion in the recovery room: A masquerader of pulmonary dysfunction. *Can J Anaesth* 1996; **43**: 1249–51.

Asai T, Koga K, Vaughn RS. Respiratory complications associated with tracheal intubation and extubation. *British Journal of Anaesthesia* 1998; **80**: 767–75.

Cooper RM. Extubation and changing endotracheal tube. In: Benumof JL, ed. Airway Management Principles and Practice. Philadelphia: Mosby, 1995.

Koga K, Asai T, Vaughan RS & Latto IP. Respiratory complications associated with tracheal extubation. Timing of tracheal extubation and use of the laryngeal mask during emergence from anaesthesia. *Anaesthesia* 1998; **53**: 540–4.

Peterson GN, Domino KB, Caplan RA, Posner KL, Lee LA, Cheney FW. Management of the difficulty airway: a closed claims analysis. *Anesthesiology* 2005; **103**: 33–9.

Practice Guidelines for Management of the Difficult Airway: An Updated Report by the American Society of Anaesthetists Task Force on Management of the Difficult Airway. *Anesthesiology* 2003; **98**: 1269–77.

Rassam S, SandbyThomas M, Vaughan RS. Airway management before, during and after extubation: a survey of practice in the United Kingdom and Ireland. *Anaesthesia* 2005; **60**: 995–1001.

Chapter 13

New airway devices for difficult airway management

Imran Ahmad and Shaun Scott

Key points

- A plethora of new airway devices has been introduced recently but not all of these are suitable for use in difficult airway scenarios
- Indirect laryngoscopes allow 'close-up' visualization of the larynx and of the intubation procedure. Though the view of the glottis is frequently better than that of direct laryngoscopes, this does not guarantee easy *intubation*
- Optical Stylets may be passed into the subglottis or held above the glottis to visualize intubation of the trachea. They can be used on their own or as an adjunct to direct laryngoscopy
- Single-use devices may be more difficult to use, be less successful and may cause increased morbidity
- It is strongly recommended that anaesthetists wishing to use any of these devices for difficult airway management first gain experience in their routine clinical practice.

13.1 Introduction

Many new airway devices have recently been introduced into anaesthesia practice. Most of those that are intended for use in difficult airway scenarios have little or no published data from patients with difficult airways. In this chapter we present and discuss some those devices that that we consider (albeit without this data) likely to be of some value. Fibreoptic and cricothyroidotomy devices are discussed elsewhere in this book.

13.2 **Indirect Laryngoscopes (IL)**

Whereas direct laryngoscopes (DL) afford a 'straight line' view of the larynx, indirect laryngoscopes conduct this image via mirrors, prisms, fibreoptic bundles, or a combination, or relay the image from a distal camera. Indirect laryngoscopes (IL) may be classified into those which incorporate a guide for the passage of a tracheal tube and those that do not (Table 13.1). LMA Ctrach® and optical stylets may be considered special cases, but are considered separately below.

IL allow a view of the glottis from a vantage point that is closer and more posterior to the larynx than during DL and should therefore be expected to provide a full view of the glottis with relative ease. However, this does not always guarantee easy *intubation*; indeed anything less than a full view may result in difficulty.

> **Box 13.1 Interpretation of view obtained by indirect laryngoscopy**
>
> • The purpose of the ideal classification grade should be to predict *ease of intubation*
>
> • No validated grading system for IL currently exists
>
> • The 'Cormack and Lehane' grade for DL is entirely unsuitable for this purpose
>
> • Studies of IL should be appraised for evidence of *intubation success* rather than mere *improvement of view*.

13.3 **Indirect Laryngoscopes with tube channel: Airtraq® and Pentax AWS®**

For pictures and video of some of these devices and their use, log on to www.orag.co.uk/book. Both of these devices are anatomically-shaped IL with a tube guide channel to the right side. This holds the tracheal tube and directs it as it is advanced by the operator. The visual axis of each scope and long axis of the tube meet at a point in front of the tip of the blade. This is brought near to the laryngeal inlet as vertical lift is applied to the device; some manipulation is required to guide the intubation under visual control.

Table 13.1 **Classification of indirect laryngoscopes**	
With tracheal tube guide	**Without tracheal tube guide**
Airtraq Optical Laryngoscope	GlideScope®Video Laryngoscpope
Pentax Airwayscope	Storz video laryngoscope
LMA Ctrach®	McGrath video laryngoscope
Optical styles	

Figure 13.1 From left, Airtraq® and Pentax-AWS®, both viewed from the right. Arrows indicate the tube channel to the right of each device

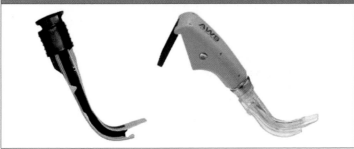

These have been shown to be easy to use and reports of successful use in difficult scenarios (obesity, failed obstetric intubation, cervical spine immobilization) are accumulating. They differ significantly in that the Pentax-AWS® must be directed into the anterior commisure while the Airtraq® is best positioned in the vallecula.

13.3.1 Airtraq® Optical Laryngoscope

The Airtraq® Optical Laryngoscope (Prodol Meditec; www.airtraq.com) is packaged individually as a single-use device and is pre-installed with batteries, powering both the distal LED light and warming the distal lens. The optical channel contains a series of plastic lenses, prisms and mirrors to transmit the image to an eyepiece that is orientated vertically on top of the handle (an optional blue-tooth camera may be attached to permit viewing on a suitable computer screen).

As a lightweight and disposable device it is potentially advantageous in awkward circumstances e.g. in the pre-hospital setting, when the operator may be forced to intubate from in front of the patient or required to wear protective clothing (limiting manual dexterity for set-up and procedure).

Box 13.2 Potential for laryngeal impingement

Indirect Laryngoscopes with tube channels:
- fixed relationship between tube axis and line of sight
- distance from glottis influences tube target
- relatively posterior approach to the glottis.

Therefore:
- impingement may occur within or about the larynx
- this may cause considerable difficulty if not anticipated.

13.3.2 Pentax-AWS

The Pentax-AWS (Airway Scope; www.pentaxmedical.com) is a reusable battery-powered indirect video-laryngoscope with built in monitor and disposable clear polycarbonate blade. The 2.4 inch LCD monitor set on a swivel-joint on the posterior aspect of the handle. The CCD camera, positioned at the distal tip of a flexible segment, is inserted into the single-use 'P-blade' which is fixed to the handle. The monitor display incorporates a 'target sight' indicating where the tube is directed (anticipated tube tip impingement to the right of the glottis, this target biases the optimal view slightly to the left).

13.4 Indirect laryngoscopes without tube guide

For pictures and techiques log on to www.orag.co.uk/book

13.4.1 GlideScope® Video Laryngoscope

The GlideScope® Video Laryngoscope (GVL®; Verathon Inc.; www.verathon. com) comprises distal high-resolution CMOS camera with anti-fogging mechanism and light-source embedded within a reusable plastic laryngoscope handle and blade, connected by a detachable cable to a small portable colour LCD monitor. The blade is slim and has a distinctive 60-degree angulation at its mid-point. The tip of the blade is advanced in the midline, positioned in the vallecula and lifted to expose the glottis, as the tracheal tube (pre-loaded with wire-stylet angulated to 60 degrees) is introduced. As the stylet is withdrawn, the tube extends and advances into the trachea. The GlideScope® Cobalt comprises a single-use version of the blade (the 'GVL Stat®') which is mounted upon a reusable 'Video Baton'.

The GlideScope® has established a role as a rescue device after difficult direct laryngoscopy and as a primary device in circumstances of anticipated difficulty. Those that are experienced in its use report high intubation success rate while novices may experience difficulty intubating the trachea in spite of accomplishing a clear view of the larynx.

13.4.2 McGrath® Video Laryngoscope

The McGrath® Series 5 video laryngoscope (Aircraft Medical Ltd; www.aircraftmedical.com) is a battery-powered portable laryngoscope with a VGA camera and 1.7 inch LCD monitor, which is mounted on a swivel at the top of its handle. The disposable clear polycarbonate blade is mounted on a steel CameraStick™ of adjustable length attached to the base of the handle. The curved, narrow profile blade (13 mm) may be negotiated into position with limited mouth opening and neck manipulation. An angulated stylet facilitates passage of the tracheal tube under visual control.

13.4.3 **Berci-Kaplan DCI® Video Laryngoscope**

The Berci-Kaplan DCI® ('Direct Coupled Interface'; Karl Storz, www.karlstorz.com) video laryngoscope range includes standard Macintosh, Dörges or Miller laryngoscope blades. The DCI® camera head and light conduit are attached within the laryngoscope handle to fibreoptic bundles in the blade, connecting the laryngoscope to a TelePack™ 12 inch LCD monitor, HiLux light source and camera control unit.

13.5 **ILMA® and Ctrach®**

The Intubating Laryngeal Mask Airway (ILMA® or LMA-Fastrach™; Intavent Orthofix www.intaventorthofix.com) has proven to be of great value not only as a primary airway management device in many *anticipated* difficult airway scenarios but also as a means of achieving secondary tracheal intubation after *unanticipated* failed direct laryngoscopy. A single-use version of the ILMA® with soft-PVC flexo-metallic tube has recently been introduced.

The LMA Ctrach® adds the advantage of indirect laryngoscopy to ILMA®, affording a view from within the mask aperture (through a modified EEB) of the larynx. This image is conducted via fibreoptic bundles to the Ctrach® Viewer (incorporating camera, 3.4' colour LCD display unit, rechargeable battery and light source) which is attached to the top of the Ctrach® stem.

13.6 **Optical Stylets**

Optical stylets are preformed with an anatomical curve, may be rigid or malleable, and some may have flexible distal segments or a working channel. They share some of the benefits of indirect laryngoscopes, namely an ability to achieve a close-up view of the larynx despite limited mouth opening or neck mobility, but have the additional advantages of providing an intubation guide that is not only in the line of sight (thus reducing the likelihood of impingement of tube tip) but that may also be advanced into the subglottis along with the tube. Whereas flexible fibrescopes are more able to negotiate around obstacles in the airway, the rigid optical stylets have the advantage of absolute control over both the orientation of the long axis and the forward force applied to the tip.

Solo (lateral 'retromolar' and midline 'sagittal') and combination (with a direct laryngoscope) techniques are described. The solo techniques require jaw and tongue lift by the non-dominant hand (or jaw thrust to be provided by an assistant) in order to gain access the larynx. When used in combination with a direct laryngoscope, which serves to lift the tongue base, the tip of the stylet and/or tube must be advanced into the subglottis before removing the laryngoscope blade, withdrawing the stylet and then advancing the tube. In this context the tube tip is best rotated to a posterior position (opposite to the fibreoptic 'railroading' technique) as it passes the cords to avoid impingement of the tip within the subglottis.

Figure 13.2 The LMA CTrach

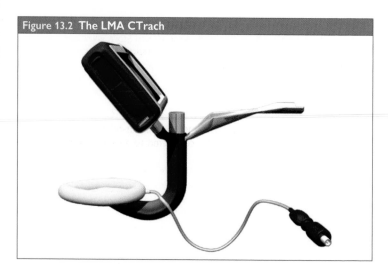

13.6.1 The Bonfils Retromolar Intubation Endoscope

Although the Bonfils (Karl Storz; www.karlstorz.com) is not a new device it has the strongest evidence base and so is included in this discussion (Figure 13.3). It is a rigid stylet of 35–40 cm length (3.5 and 5.0 mm outer diameter, respectively) with a 40-degree curvature of the distal tip; the larger version contains a 1.2 mm i.d. working channel. The image resolution is of high-quality with 35,000 pixels. It is available in two formats: eyepiece (housed atop the handle, hinged in the sagittal plane) and DCI®. The DCI® version may be converted to a portable device with an eyepiece attachment and battery-powered light-source.

Figure 13.3 The Bonfils Retromolar Intubation Endoscope

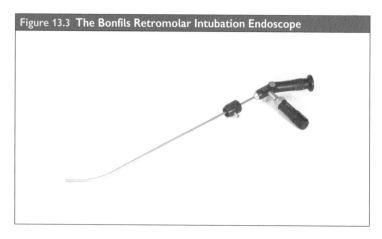

13.6.2 **The SensaScope**

The SensaScope (Acutronic MS, Hirzel, Switzerland; acutronic-medical.ch) is a guidable fibreoptic stylet 43 cm long and 6.0 mm outer diameter. The rigid part of the stylet has an S-shaped curve while the 3 cm-long steerable tip (bending 60 degrees up/down), is controlled by a conventional thumb-lever on the handle.

13.6.3 **The Levitan FPS Scope and Shikani Optical Stylet 'SOS™'**

The Levitan FPS ('First Pass Success') and Shikani Optical Stylet (both manufactured by Clarus Medical Systems; www.clarus-medical.com) comprise a semi-rigid malleable fibreoptic stylet connected to an eyepiece and battery-powered light source.

The Shikani has a 40cm stylet, while the Levitan FPS is 30 cm, which matches more closely the length of the endotracheal tube, making it easier for the operator to reach the eyepiece and allowing for easier manipulation of the tip of the stylet. The stylet tip should be angulated to about 35 degrees when used in conjunction with a direct laryngoscope, and 70 degrees when used as a solo device. They are powered by a specific light-weight battery-pack (conveniently, the Levitan may connect to a laryngoscope handle).

Figure 13.4 **The Bonfils, SensaScope and Levitan FPS optical stylets**

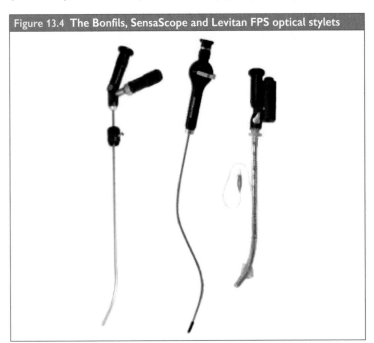

Box 13.3 **Advantages and disadvantages of indirect laryngoscopes and optical stylets**

Advantages:
- more easily obtain full view of the larynx
- permit close visualization of tube entering glottis, and/or provides 'railroad' into trachea.

Disadvantages:
- the view may be obscured by blood or secretions on the distal lens
- intubation may be difficult despite clear view of larynx
- nasotracheal intubation may be observed but not facilitated
- no inspection of the lower airway possible.

13.7 **Single-use bougies**

While the reusable Eschmann Tracheal Tube Introducer ('gum-elastic bougie'; SIMS-Portex) remains the current gold-standard intubation aid, a number of single-use alternatives are now available with satisfactory rigidity and ability to retain a chosen curvature. Moreover, several are produced with distal side-holes, a lumen, and means for proximal connection of gas sampling-line or an insufflator. When in doubt after difficult direct laryngoscopy and introducer-placement, it is possible to confirm tracheal placement by measurement of end-tidal carbon dioxide (a single chest compression may be required to expel carbon dioxide into the trachea of the apnoeic patient, to prevent a false-negative result) or to administer oxygen if tube passage is delayed. Although it is possible to attach the capnometry sampling line prior to intubation if the situation is anticipated to be difficult, this necessitates pre-loading of the endotracheal tube (or a second assistant) if cricoid pressure is to be maintained by the first assistant during a rapid-sequence induction.

13.7.1 **The Multi-function Intubating Bougie**

('MIB'; BreatheSafe®, OGM Ltd; www.breathesafe.uk.com) is a composite of two plastic tubes: the inner is firm and malleable while the outer is soft with a low-friction satin finish. It is necessary for the user to fashion a coudé tip and oro-pharyngeal curve from the straight MIB prior to use. The soft tip contains four distal side-holes while the proximal end has an integral low-profile Luer slip connector.

13.7.2 **The Frova Intubating Introducer**

(Cook Medical Inc; www.cookmedical.com) is straight with a preformed coudé tip with rounded atraumatic end containing two lateral side holes. It is hollow along its length, allowing the passage of an optional wire 'stiffening cannula'. Also optional is the 'Rapi-Fit Adapter' (without which Luer connection is not possible).

13.8 Supraglottic devices

A multitude of new supraglottic airway devices have entered the market recently. Many of these are meritorious and some appear to have potential to be of use in the management of the difficult airway.

13.8.1 Pro-Seal® LMA

The Pro-Seal® LMA (LMA Company; lmaco.com) was introduced in the UK in 2001. Compared to the LMA Classic® (cLMA) it has a softer, larger bowl, an additional dorsal cuff, a drainage tube running parallel to the airway tube and an integral bite block. These changes allow an improved peri-laryngeal seal, a reduction in the likelihood of gastric inflation and increased protection from aspiration if regurgitation occurs. Its use has been recommended after unanticipated difficult intubation in the rapid sequence induction scenario, where there is a need to continue emergency surgery.

13.8.2 LMA Supreme

The LMA Supreme™ (LMA Company; lmaco.com) is the most recent introduction to the LMA family. It is disposable and available in three adult sizes. The enlarged cuff enhances anatomical fit and the reinforcing tip prevents folding-over of the mask. It has a semi-rigid, anatomically-curved airway tube (similar to ILMA) allowing easy insertion. The airway tube is elliptical in cross-section with an integral bite block, a kink-resistant lateral groove and a drainage tube. 'Epiglottic fins' are intended to prevent the epiglottis from obstructing the airway.

13.8.3 i-gel

The i-gel (Intersurgical Ltd, www.i-gel.com) is a novel supraglottic airway device with a non-inflatable 'cuff' made of a soft thermoplastic elastomer. It is for single patient use and is available in three adult sizes. It has a short, wide stem (with integral bite-block) which provides a suitable conduit for secondary intubation with a fibrescope – when compared with cLMA, the i-gel will allow tubes of larger diameter to pass through its airway tube. The larger (therefore longer) endotracheal tube will consequently protrude further from the (shorter) stem of the i-gel, permitting the tube cuff to pass beyond the vocal cords.

Further reading

Cooper R.M., Pacey J.A., Bishop M.J., McCluskey S.A. Early experience with a new videolaryngoscope (Glidescope) in 728 patients. *Can J Anaes* 2005; **52**: 191–8.

Hagberg C.A. (2007) Current concepts in the management of the difficult airway. *Anesthesiology News*, 2007; May, 1–19.

Halligan M. and Charters P. A clinical evaluation of the Bonfils Intubation Fibrescope. *Anaesthesia 2003*; **58**: 1087–91.

Levitan R.M. Design rationale and intended use of a short optical stylet for routine fibreoptic augmentation of emergency laryngoscopy. *Am J Emerg Med* 2006; **24**: 490–5.

Maharaj C.H., Costello J.F., Harte B.H., Laffey J.G. (2008). Evaluation of the Airtraq and Macintosh laryngoscopes in patients at increased risk for difficult tracheal intubation. *Anaesthesia* 2007; **63**: 182–8.

Mihai R., Blair E., Kay H., Cook T.M. A quantitative review and meta-analysis of performance of non-standard laryngoscopes and rigid fibreoptic intubation aids. *Anaesthesia 2008;* **63**: 745–60.

Suzuki A., Toyama Y., Katsumi N. *et al* The Pentax-AWS® rigid indirect video laryngoscope: clinical assessment of performance in 320 cases. *Anaesthesia 2008.* **63**: 641–7.

Timmermann A., Russo S. and Graf B.M.. Evaluation of the CTrach- an intubating LMA with integrated fibreoptic system. *Br J Anaesth* 2006; **96**: 516–21.

Chapter 14

Airway training

Imogen Davies and Mansukh Popat

Key points

- The aim of airway training must be to provide (trainee) anaesthetists with the knowledge, behaviour, and practical skills that they can use effectively and reliably to maintain oxygenation of a patient
- Training in airway management should ensure that anaesthetists are at least able to gain competencies recommended in guidelines appropriate to their country
- To achieve these aims, a structured approach to airway training using an 'off patient' and 'on patient' model is suggested
- Each department should be able to provide this 'off patient' training locally. An Airway Training Room equipped with dedicated equipment for training is mandatory
- On patient training requires experienced trainers, targeted operating lists and dedicated equipment.
- A dedicated 'block rotation' in airway training maximizes training opportunities. Currently this is available in only 20% of UK departments
- Surveys reveal a serious deficiency in airway training, (especially of advanced techniques) in the UK. This situation needs to be rectified urgently.

14.1 What is training?

Training and learning describe different facets of a process which results in a change of behaviour. To change behaviour, the learner needs to change their attitude and thinking towards a subject, so airway training should endeavour to change the way a learner approaches the whole topic of airway managemant.

14.2 **Why do we need airway training?**

The aim of airway training must be to provide (trainee) anaesthetists with the knowledge, behaviour, and practical skills that they can use effectively and reliably to maintain oxygenation of a patient.

Closed claims data in the USA and Confidential Reports of maternal mortality in the UK suggest airway complications as a major cause of anaesthetic morbidity and mortality (Chapter 1). Further analysis reveals that lack of practical (advanced) skills and human behavioural factors are responsible.

This is what happens........

Knowledge: We are constantly taught that predicting a 'difficult' airway is not an exact science.

Behaviour: Therefore we either avoid performing a pre-operative airway assessment or ignore findings if these suggest that 'difficulties' may arise. We have a belief that a 'can't ventilate' scenario is rare and can't happen to us.

Skills: We therefore use high risk airway strategies especially multiple attempts at direct laryngoscopy in the paralysed patient.

This is what should happen if we wish to practice safe airway management

Knowledge: We have to accept that predicting a 'difficult' airway is not an exact science.

Behaviour: Despite this we should perform pre-operative assessment because it allows us to 'think' difficult if tests are not normal. We are therefore better prepared for the unexpected difficult airway 'can't ventilate' scenario.

Skills: Learn and practice 'low risk strategies' especially alternatives to direct laryngoscopy and awake intubation.

14.3 **What should we teach?**

We need to recognize that airway management begins with the pre-operative assessment and ends with the post-operative patient awake, spontaneously breathing, and oxygenated in recovery. All parts of this process need to be taught with the appropriate knowledge, behaviour, and practical skills.

In the UK, the Royal College of Anaesthetists (RCoA) publishes the syllabus for Competency Based Training. The Difficult Airway Society in the UK has published guidelines for the management of the unanticipated difficult airway-other countries have their equivalents. Training in airway management should ensure that anaesthetists are at least able to follow the guidelines appropriate to their country. To do this, they need to know them and be able to perform the skills contained in them.

Competency based airway training can be provided by identifying broad aims.

For example, for Basic Level (ST1/ST2) trainees the *aim* should be that they are able to

- intubate Cormack and Lehane grade I & II patients;
- effect a range of rescue manoeuvres to *optimize* attempts at intubation;
- use a bougie effectively;
- recognize a failed intubation;
- prioritize oxygenation and ventilation over intubation.

The *aims* can then be broken down into the following objectives:

Knowledge:	e.g. pre operative airway assessment, theoretical aspects of equipment (laryngoscopes, bougie) and techniques
Behaviour:	How to recognize failed intubation, when to stop attempts at intubation, when to call for help.
Skills:	Face mask ventilation, optimum technique of direct laryngoscopy with Macintosh blade, use of bougie, use of alternative laryngoscopes (McCoy/Straight blade).

All the above are 'basic' skills and facilitate Plan A of the DAS algorithm (Chapter 8).

At a later stage – during intermediate training (ST3/4) trainees could be introduced to the more 'advanced' skills to implement plans B and C of the DAS algorithm. Plan B skills would include fibreoptic assisted intubation through the LMA/ILMA and plan C would include awake fibreoptic intubation.

The above scheme is just one example of the way in which structured airway training can be provided. The syllabus needs to be comprehensive with defined aims and objectives for a number of airway scenarios so that knowledge, behaviour, and skills can be identified for each and taught appropriately.

14.4 How should we provide airway training?

Some of the skills listed are 'basic', e.g. face mask ventilation, LMA insertion, optimized direct laryngoscopy. These skills can and should be taught by every consultant trainer because they do not require any special equipment or training methods. It is important that trainees actively seek to increase numbers especially of face mask ventilation and tracheal intubation.

Use of LMA, ILMA for fibreoptic intubation, oral/nasal fibreoptic intubation and other 'advanced' techniques require a different approach. Yet some others such as cricothyroidotomy are not routinely performed on patients and therefore require training on manikins/simulators. A structured approach to facilitate training is therefore required and includes:

1. Off Patient Training
   a) Knowledge teaching
   b) Models and manikins
   c) Simulators
2. On Patient Training
   a) Trained and experienced trainers
   b) Co-operative Hospital Trusts and Departments

14.4.1 **Off Patient Training**

Most of the advanced airway techniques mentioned are complex and require a thorough understanding of equipment and execution of technique with good manual dexterity skills. A step by step approach is recommended.

14.4.1.1 *Knowledge Teaching*

Facts can be learnt at a superficial or deep level. Deep learning means that the facts have been integrated into the trainees' thinking, so that they make sense and can be applied in future situations that are unfamiliar.

Methods of acquiring knowledge at a deep, integrated level vary between learners. Some methods which may be effective by stimulating discussion and integrating new information into a trainee's existing knowledge base and experience include:

- tutorials, discussion groups
- interactive videos and CDs
- one to one or group teaching.

14.4.1.2 *Skills Teaching on Models and Manikins*

For pictures of some models used for fibreoptic training, log on to www.orag.co.uk/book

Several models of the 'hit the hole' variety have been developed to understand and improve manipulation skills with the flexible fibreoptic scope. An example is the Oxford Fibreoptic Training Box which is light-weight, portable, easy to use and has been shown to improve manual dexterity skills which are transferable to the operating room.

Manikins are useful to demonstrate and practice steps of various techniques. There is no pressure on time and no patient safety or ethical issues to worry about. The disadvantages are that even the best manikins do not mimic the human anatomy exactly, nor do they provide the challenges of blood and secretions.

14.4.1.3 *Simulators*

High fidelity simulators have the capability to mimic some of the difficult airway scenarios. They can provide real time responses to interventions and allow team behaviour to be practiced and scored. They are best used to train for unlikely scenarios involving team work or a complicated set of individual skills that have to be integrated to provide effective management of the situation, e.g. unanticipated difficult intubation. An additional advantage is that they usually include cameras so that the scenario can be taped and used for feedback. However, they are expensive to buy and require a large number of faculty who are able and willing to run them.

There are several workshops available nationally in the UK that provide the type of 'off patient' airway training mentioned. However, these are not of much benefit if the learnt techniques are not practiced subsequently on patients in the operating theatre. It is therefore vital that each department is able to provide this 'off patient' training locally. An Airway Training Room equipped with dedicated equipment for training is mandatory.

14.4.2 **On Patient Training**

It is mandatory to undergo the 'off patient' training described before being trained on patients. The training should be provided by trainers who themselves have experience of performing the techniques they wish to teach, are using these techniques routinely and have access to the required equipment and assistance. This is why the operating lists need to be 'targeted'. One trainer cannot provide training in all the techniques and a department would need several training lists with several trainers designated to provide specified training.

Consideration of the issues relating to training in advanced airway techniques has resulted in a debate about consent. In the UK, the AAGBI recommends at least verbal consent for anaesthesia but not for each individual anaesthetic procedure, so long as it is performed *routinely*. It draws attention to the risk of restricted consent whereby a patient may give consent for anaesthesia but not for intubation.

This implies that no specific consent is required as long as the advanced airway technique (such as fibreoptic intubation) that a trainer teaches is part of his/her routine practice. This approach puts the issue of teaching advanced airway techniques on the same basis as other routine techniques such as regional block and invasive monitoring procedures.

It has been shown that training can be maximized if the combined 'off patient' and 'on patient' training is provided as a 'block' rotation i.e. assigning trainees to a dedicated 'Airway Management' training module for a defined period of time.

14.5 **What is the current state of airway training in the UK?**

Literature data suggests that the 'block rotation' training mentioned above is offered in the UK in only about 20% of the departments compared to the USA (35%) and Canada (28%). Almost all departments that provide 'Block training' provide a structured programme in learning fibreoptic intubation. Several audits of availability of airway training presented at annual DAS meetings suggest that there is deficiency in all aspects of airway training. For example, a significant proportion of anaesthetists do not know what 'hold up' is (described in the Difficult Airway Society Guidelines for correct insertion of bougie) nor do many anaesthetists know where their emergency jet ventilator device is stored. When trainees were surveyed, 94% responded that they considered Awake Fibreoptic Intubation (AFI) as a core skill and needed at least 10 AFI to be competent. Yet the median number actually performed was only two AFI by the time trainees completed their training. Data has also shown that there is a geographical variation in availability of advanced airway training especially fibreoptic intubation. This reinforces the concept of agreeing 'core skills' and the minimum number to be performed competently by trainees before they are signed off.

14.6 Why is airway training so poor?

The reasons are multifactoral:

Organizational: In the UK the RCoA is responsible for defining the syllabus for the competency based training. A well structured module with defined airway competencies exits for the initial test of competency in the first year of training. Further in the training, for example in intermediate training (ST 3/4), airway competencies are grouped in with the other competencies and not as a dedicated module.

Lack of training time: Although the total time spent in anaesthesia training has not changed, due to European Working time Directive (EWTD), trainees spent far less time actually being trained. Requirement to cover obstetrics and Intensive Care also reduce the time spent in theatres.

Change in clinical practice: The number of intubations and face mask anesthesia cases have markedly dropped since the routine use of supraglottic devices.

Lack of trainers: Contrary to popular belief lack of equipment and operating lists is not a problem. However, there is a problem matching able and willing trainers with willing trainees.

14.7 How can we improve airway training?

Specific airway skills training, at nationally advertised courses or workshops can help increase the trainee's knowledge of different techniques but much of the basic airway assessment and management must be taught in the trainee's own department.

Training must be targeted. Within a department, lists which are known to have airway training opportunities (challenging intubations, cases for facemask anaesthesia or uncommon anaesthesia methods such as jet ventilation) should never be without at least one trainee. Having a team of consultant, senior trainee and junior trainee allows the senior to teach the junior trainee more basic skills and then the consultant to teach the senior. This method of not losing training opportunities requires the cooperation of the departmental rota-writer, consultants and trainees.

The Hospital Trust or School of Anaesthesia should recognize the importance of 'off patient' training and provide a training room and equipment for in house airway workshops. This would be greatly facilitated if an 'Airway Training Co-ordinator' was appointed for each department.

There needs to be recognition that modern airway training requires a structured approach: there is an urgent need to identify 'core airway' skills that all trainees should be taught and assessed as competent in. One way to do this is by introducing the structured approach discussed.

Further reading

Cook TM. (Still) time to organise training in airway management in UK. *Anaesthesia* 2006; **61**: 727–30.

Cooper G. Is the art of airway management being lost? *BJA CEPD Reviews;* **2**: 662–3.

Hegberg CA, Greger J, Chelly JE, Saa-Eddin HE. Instruction of Airway Management Skills During Anesthesiology Residency Training. *Journal of Clinical Anesthesia* 2003; **15**: 149–53.

Kiyama S, Muthuswamy D, Latto IP, Asai T. Prevalence of a training module for difficult airway management: A comparison between Japan and the United Kingdom. *Anaesthesia* 2003; **58**: 571–3.

Koppel JN, Reed AP. Formal instruction in difficult airway management: a survey of Anesthesiology Residency programs. *Anesthesiology* 1995; **83**: 1343–6.

McNarry AF, Dovell T, Dancey FM, Pead ME. Perception of training needs and opportunities in advanced airway skills: a survey of British and Irish trainees. *Eur J Anaesthesiol.* **2007**: 498–504.

Mohanna, K, Wall, D, Chambers, R. *Teaching Made Easy.* Radcliffe Medical Press Second Edition, 2004.

Popat M. State of the art – The Airway (editorial). *Anaesthesia* 2003; **58**: 1166–70.

Rosenblatt WH, Wagner PJ, Ovassapian A, Kain ZN. Practice patterns in managing the difficult airway by anaesthetists in the United States. *Anesthesia and Analgesia* 1998; **87**: 153–7.

Stringer KR, Bajenov S, Yentis SM. Training in airway management. *Anaesthesia* 2002; **57**: 967–98.

Index

C